FeD UP
With Being
FAT & SICK

by
Judith Fiore, BA, ND
and
Diane McConnell, BA, BT

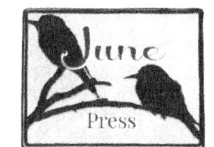

Copy right © 2017
All rights reserved

Judith Fiore & Diane McConnell

Disclaimer:

In this book, *Fed Up with Being Fat and Sick*, you are going to hear about a lot of people who have cured their chronic diseases and lost large amounts of weight by following the eating plan outlined here. Although you can expect improvements in your health, as well as weight loss, you agree to accept full responsibility for your own health and success. There is no guarantee that what has worked for the people that have been interviewed for this book will also work for you. Your body and circumstances are unique to you. You accept full responsibility for the use and misuse of the information contained in this book. Any results that you achieve are entirely due to your own effort. For all illnesses, we do strongly recommend that you consult with a physician, particularly if you are currently under the care of a medical practitioner and are undergoing treatments and/or taking prescribed medications.

Dedication

Judith Fiore & Diane McConnell

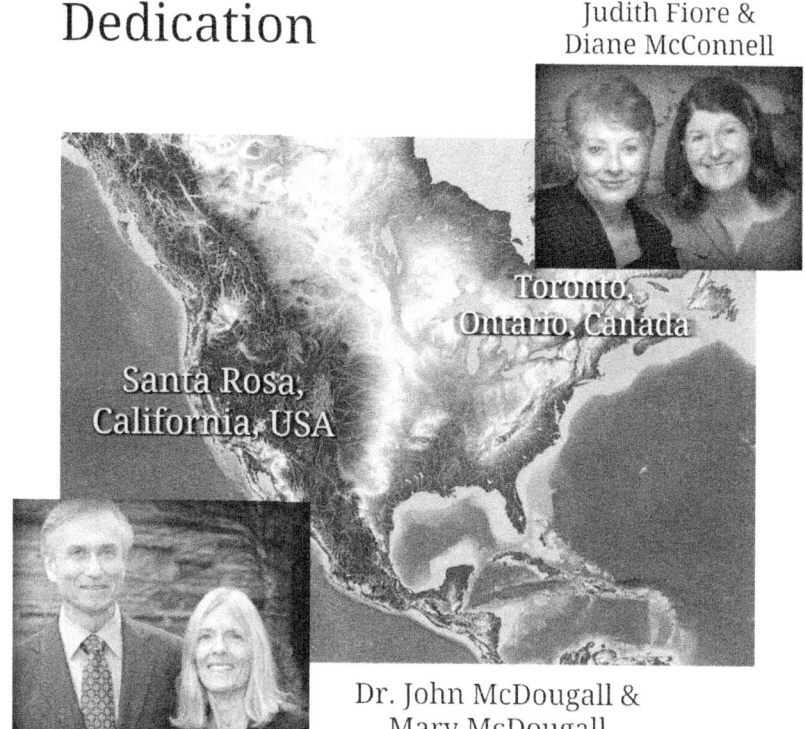

Toronto, Ontario, Canada

Santa Rosa, California, USA

Dr. John McDougall & Mary McDougall

We dedicate this book to our two heroes, Dr. John McDougall and Mary McDougall from Santa Rosa, California. Even from the distance of 2,645 miles, the impact of your life's work has profoundly changed and improved the quality of our lives here in Toronto. Our health has been restored. It is with deep respect and appreciation that our hearts reach out to your hearts. Thank you for everything that you have done to spread the truth about healthy eating.

Toronto Starch Solution Meetup Group
Group Toronto Starch Solution Meetup

Acknowledgments

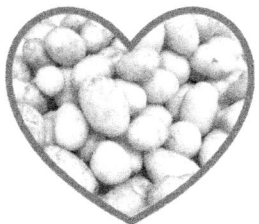

This book could not have happened without acknowledging the incredible work and dedication of the following health care advocates that we look up to and admire: Michael Greger, MD; Caldwell Esselstyn, MD; Neal Barnard, MD; T. Colin Campbell, PhD; Douglas Lisle, PhD; Alan Goldhamer, DC; Joel Fuhrman, MD; Richard Oppenlander, DDS; Jeff Novick, RD; Brenda Davis, RD; Julieanna Hever, RD; Chef AJ; John Pierre and of course the man we most subscribe to: John McDougall, MD and his amazing wife Mary McDougall. A huge bunch of thanks to all these wonderful men and women. They are our heroes.

This publication would not be complete without the interviews of Dr. John McDougall, Amy Tan, Lori and Murray Nichol, Cecilia Burke, Judy Newman, Dom Fiore, Sabina Poirier, Carol and Dan Farr, and Jane Caddick. A heartfelt thanks to all of you.

Additionally, we would like to thank Rose Oliva and Judy Newman for their fantastic editing skills. Their input has given this book the final polish it needed.

We'd like to acknowledge the support of Dom Fiore, Juliana Fiore, and Lorne McConnell for being there, as well as members of the Toronto Starch Solution Meet up group – in particular, Kathy, Tom and Petra, three of our founding members.

We are also very grateful to the Don Heights Unitarian Church for providing us with a wonderful space
to host our monthly potluck meetings.

And finally to our wonderful dogs, Lulu and Zero. They make our lives so much better and brighter.

Toronto Starch Solution Meetup Group
Group Toronto Starch Solution Meetup

Table of Contents

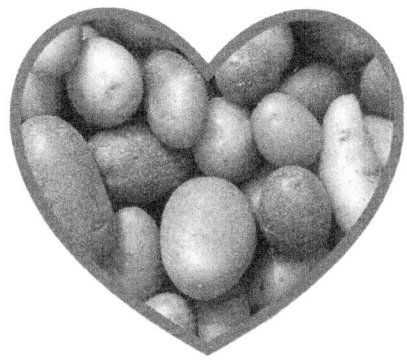

Toronto Starch Solution Meetup Group
Group Toronto Starch Solution Meetup

Table of Contents

Introduction by Judith Fiore, ND 2

Chapter One - The Starchivore Paradigm 6

Chapter Two - Dr. John McDougall's Interview 16

Chapter Three - McDougall's McFACTS 44

Chapter Four - Dr. John McDougall's Program 64

Chapter Five - Amy's Interview 80

Chapter Six - Diane's Interview 94

Chapter Seven - Lori's Interview 112

Chapter Eight - Judy's Interview 136

Chapter Nine - Jane's Interview 158

Chapter Ten - Carol's Interview 174

Chapter Eleven - Dan's Interview 188

Chapter Twelve - Cecilia's Interview 202

Chapter Thirteen - Sabina's Interview 216

Chapter Fourteen - Judith's Interview 234

Chapter Fifteen - Dom's Interview 252

Chapter Sixteen - Murray's Interview 268

A Last Word from Diane McConnell 282

References 286

Resources 300

Introduction

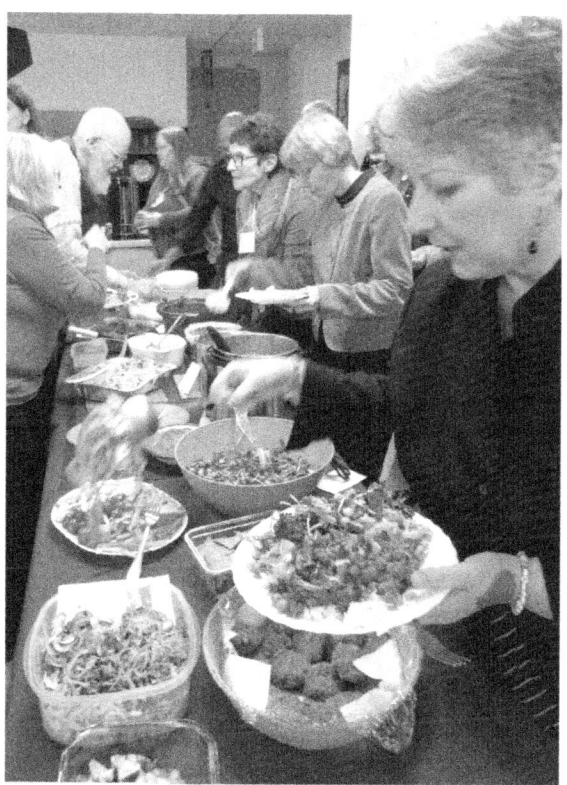

Toronto Starch Solution Meetup Group
Group Toronto Starch Solution Meetup

Judith Fiore & Diane McConnell

Introduction by Judith Fiore, ND

These are the stories of a group of middle-aged folks from Toronto who learned about Dr. John McDougall and the power of a whole food plant-based, starch-centered way of eating. We were dealing with too much weight, high cholesterol, diabetes, high blood pressure, arthritis, lupus, and cardiovascular disease. Our lives were going in the same direction as most people who develop health issues in their 40s, 50s, and 60s. We were taking pills to lower blood pressure, cholesterol, and blood sugar; pills to manage arthritic flare ups, and more pills to deal with the pain. There were even pills to treat the side effects from all the other pills. The only direction that we could eventually see in our future was one in which we would lose our health and go to our graves at least 10 years before we should.

Diane and I decided we wanted to write this book for anyone who needs to be inspired by the stories of other regular people, and who is looking for an effective, nutritional way to lose excess weight and get healthy. Our hope is that our experiences with the McDougall way of eating will encourage you to change how you're eating, and most likely, improve your health and your life. We believe that for many of you, these stories could inspire you to save your life. In chapters one and four, we've included some guidance on following Dr. McDougall's plan, written from the point of view of people who have experienced profound improvements in health as well as shrinking waist lines.

The Toronto Starch Solution group began in October 2015. I had been on the McDougall forum, and I was hoping to meet at least one other starchivore in Toronto. I wanted a chance to get together at least monthly, share recipe ideas, and support and encourage one another. I found Judy and Kathy, who had also been trying to set up regular meetings. It was proving to be a difficult thing, getting people to commit to face-to-face support.

When Judy, Kathy, and I sat down together at our first meeting, it was exciting to share each other's stories, and talk freely about how we were improving our health. We came up with the idea of a Meetup group where we could attract other starchivores. That was when The Toronto Starch Solution Meetup group was born. By the next meeting, we were seven people. Judy offered her church as a monthly meeting place where we could hold potlucks, have speakers, and show videos and films. Over time, our membership has grown to over 150 people, and we're still growing.

The monthly potlucks are a wonderful opportunity for us to get together for fellowship and education. The food is simply glorious. We eat chili, sushi, shepherd's pie, soup, stew, stir fry, lasagna, banana bread, cookies, and a lot more. Oh, and there's usually salad and fruit. It is an amazing spread, and it exemplifies the incredible variety and deliciousness of eating an oil-free, whole food diet that is starch-centered and devoid of all animal products. We can't imagine eating any other way. Our lives have been vastly improved, and we are grateful for the support we're receiving from one another, and for Dr. McDougall's many years of promoting this way of eating.

Although the terms starch-centered and plant-based are primarily used throughout this book, it is important to confirm that Dr. McDougall's preferred term "starch-based" is the most correct and useful way to refer to this way of eating. As you read through the first chapters that describe his starch-based plan, and read the interviews of members of our Toronto Starch Solution Meetup group, keep in mind that our better health is due to eating starches like potatoes, whole intact grains, squashes, beans, chickpeas, and lentils. They're all plant foods, but more importantly, they're all starches.

This book is a tribute to Dr. John McDougall and his wife Mary, and to our fellow members of the Toronto Starch Solution Meetup group. We hope you are inspired by our stories, and the sound, science-based

Judith Fiore & Diane McConnell

advice we are sharing that has helped us regain our health. It's not about willpower, it's about eating the right kind of food, the starch-based food that we humans are meant to thrive on.

Toronto, Ontario

July 28th, 2017

Chapter One
The Starchivore Paradigm

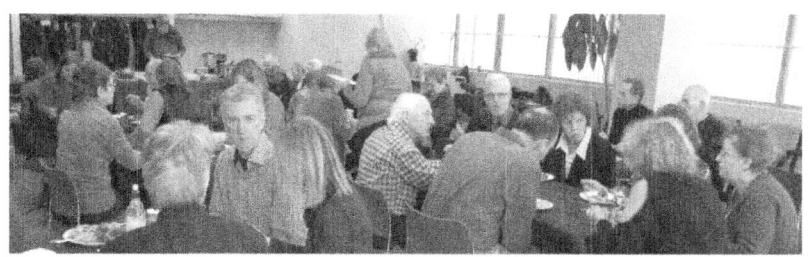

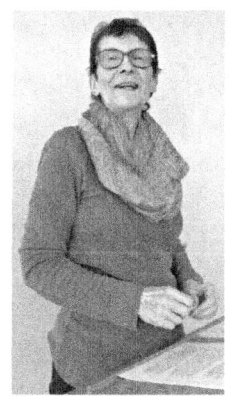
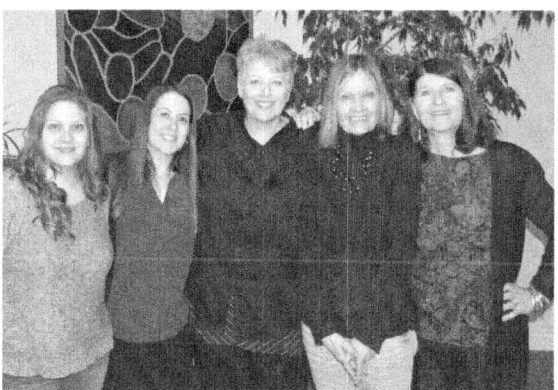

Toronto Starch Solution Meetup Group
Group Toronto Starch Solution Meetup

Chapter One - The Starchivore Paradigm

The world is in a health crisis. There are 2.1 billion overweight people in the world.[1,2] It is now close to one-third of our world population that is obese or overweight according to statistics from the data of 188 countries. Of these, 312 million are obese.[1,2] A staggering 18 million people are going to die this year of heart disease and 18 million more next year.3 In 2014, it was reported that 422 million people worldwide had diabetes.[4] It is also estimated that 40 percent of all people who eat the standard American diet will develop cancer.[5-7] These illnesses: heart disease, type 2 diabetes, and cancer, are preventable and reversible in the vast majority by simply eating a whole food, plant-based diet that is oil-free.[8,9]

Nutritional science has come a long way. Research on how a whole food, plant-based diet is reversing and preventing disease is very persuasive. Let's face it, the health of the average 60 year-old isn't exactly stellar. When you look at what most people in their 60s are eating, and then look at what the research is saying, it's no surprise that getting older is usually fraught with pills and procedures. We are killing ourselves by indulging daily in animal foods. As Dr. McDougall says, animal foods are poison.[10-12] It's time to stop poisoning yourself. It's time to take this incredible opportunity to take responsibility for your health and feel good again.

In the introduction to his brilliant book, *The Starch Solution*[13], Dr. John McDougall shares that he has often been asked why he, as a doctor, speaks against the practices of his colleagues. His reply is simply that he never took the Hippocratic oath to protect the financial interests of the medical industry. Instead, the oath he took asked him to care for the sick and keep them from harm and injustice. This means never giving patients a deadly drug or procedure. Dr. McDougall knows that his views cause those with vested interests to dislike him. He has made his peace with the criticisms. Unfortunately, too many physicians and dietitians fall in line with the interests of the food and pharmaceutical industries over the needs of their patients. Dr. McDougall believes that his colleagues are well intentioned, but their lack of knowledge of basic human nutrition prevents them from being able to heal their patients and protect them from harm.[14]

Dr. McDougall has written several books on preventing and reversing serious disease through a low-fat, starch-centered diet. The book that brought our group together is *The Starch Solution, Eat the Foods You Love, Regain Your Health, and Lose the Weight for Good!*[13] There is a picture of a potato on the cover. Anyone who thinks weight loss depends on getting rid of all carbs, including potatoes, would be in for a surprise. This way of eating asks that you eat those potatoes, in fact, to please eat all kinds of potatoes. You also eat oatmeal, brown rice, buckwheat, quinoa, and a wide variety of squashes.

For those of us with weight issues, our doctors would admonish us for not being able to lose weight. Very often we heard the words, "If you could lose this weight many of your health problems would go away." This is true. If a person is at a normal weight, there are fewer worries with high blood pressure and diabetes. But there are many who are not overweight and who are stricken with disease and debilitation too. It is not always a straightforward solution, losing weight and expecting to lose the disease we suffer from.

Taking the nutritional route means you are in control. You have the power to get better, just by what you choose to put on your plate. It really is your choice, even if you have strong cravings for animal foods, fried foods, and dairy foods like ice cream and cheese. Those cravings are powerful, there's no denying that. We have found that by sticking to a low-fat, whole food starch-centered diet, in time, the cravings diminish. When you know that eating those foods increases your blood pressure or causes an attack of arthritis, it can be a further incentive to choose to eat the foods that will not harm you. It's a choice that will help you feel better and add years of quality living to your life.

For some of you who are fortunate to not be facing a serious health issue but are overweight, then following a starch-centered diet is going to be an amazing thing. Weight loss is almost effortless. You never go hungry. You eat until you are satisfied. There are no calories or points to count, no glycemic index tables to fret over, and you can enjoy a wide range of foods. If you're tired of being fat, then you have a simple and beautiful plan to finally get rid of the weight and look and feel better.

Speaking of looking and feeling better, there is an increase in energy when eating a starch-centered, oil-free diet. If you are feeling less than enthusiastic about exercise, once you begin this way of eating you will probably find you've acquired an extra gear. Before you know it, you will want to move your body. If you enjoy walking, as you lose weight and regain your health, you'll be walking at a brisker pace and for longer distances. The same for other activities like swimming or cycling. You may also find you prefer to take the stairs instead of the elevator. The shocking thing is that exercise may become something you do for enjoyment and not to punish yourself!

The Lure of Sugar, Salt, and Fat

The Standard American Diet (SAD) is probably the leading cause of chronic illness and premature death.[15, 16] The SAD way of eating is what we grew up on and believed was healthy. Sadly, all those years of loading our plates with meats, dairy, fish, eggs, oils, butter, and large portions of refined carbohydrates like breads, pasta, cookies, cakes, doughnuts, and other junk foods, have led us to being fat, sick, tired, and hungry. Obesity rates are climbing, along with the numbers of people diagnosed with diabetes, heart disease, and cancer.[16] We were raised to believe that the good life means eating large portions of fatty and fried foods. It's easy to remember as teenagers, how meeting friends at the local café for fries and gravy was a Saturday highlight. If there were a few extra dollars, butterscotch sundaes were sure to be ordered. It was an afternoon of pure indulgence over fatty, salty, and sugary foods.

What many people don't realize is that a steady diet of high fat foods, especially when processed with salt and sugar, does something to our brains. There has been a considerable amount of nutritional research on how eating fatty, salty, and sugary foods lead to addictive behavior.[17] For many of us, once we start, we want to keep eating more and more of those foods because the pleasure centers of our brains are wired to want more and more of those foods. In fact, it has been shown that obese adults, who are not alcoholics or drug addicts, have the same genetic marker that is found with alcoholism and other drug addictions.[17]

In addition, it's been shown that we humans produce opioids when we eat excess sugars and fats.[18] In fact, there's been research showing that obese adults have a physical craving for fatty and sugary foods. In one study, when obese subjects were given naloxone, an opiate blocker, they lost interest in eating sugary, fatty foods like candies and cookies.[19] This kind of research shows that sugary, fatty foods stimulate the pleasure centers of the brain.

In their book, *The Pleasure Trap*, Dr. Douglas Lisle and Dr. Alan Goldhamer write about how important it is for a species to seek out pleasure and avoid pain in order to survive.[20] The reward for seeking out pleasure is to eat enough to see us through times of little food, as well as seeking out a mate and making babies. The problem for people in the West is that we have a huge amount of pleasure-inducing foods being marketed to us day in and day out. We turn on our television sets, and there they are, those commercials with seductive close-ups of foods that feature fat, salt, and sugar. You don't even have to be hungry to start thinking, "Oh, pizza would be nice. Oh, I still have some ice cream in the fridge, and isn't there some left over fried chicken?" We are bombarded with temptations just driving down the street, hence the drive-through convenience of picking up a greasy, salty burger and fries, all washed down with a sugary soda pop or milkshake.

It's estimated that about two-thirds of people are susceptible to food addiction, or at least strong cravings for the foods that feature the unholy triad of sugar, salt, and fat.[17-19] In the West, the estimate for the number of people who are overweight or obese is about two-thirds of the population. No surprise there, if two-thirds of us have the genetic tendency to become addicted to foods high in sugar, salt, and fat, then it is a simple correlation to link the genetics with the number of people who have a weight problem.[17-19]

Making the Change

In the past 30 years, nutritional research has been showing how a plant-based diet improves health, and how diets high in meats, dairy, and eggs are killing us.[5-13] Due to the lack of information and education, it has become a common belief that illnesses like heart disease, cancer, and diabetes are just a part of getting older. Yet, in almost every person who adopts a no-oil, plant-based diet, those life-threatening illnesses are resolved.[8, 13, 21, 22] Heart disease is reversed, diabetes and arthritis go away, and cancer may go into remission. If you are suffering from a disease that you believe is going to kill you, you owe it to yourself to take charge and start eating the kinds of foods that will probably save your life.

Even though we find this program to be a simple and beautiful way to eat, it isn't the easiest change to make. You will be letting go of many foods that you grew up with, and that you love to eat. You're probably addicted to those foods, and it can be a physically difficult road to follow. It can be socially isolating too, especially if you undertake this without support and fellowship. We are social creatures, we love to socialize over meals, and we do it a lot. If we want to get together with friends and family, it's often over a meal, a backyard barbecue, or a night out at a favorite restaurant. How do we cope when we take away the foods that have always brought us together?

The answer is we simply change the recipes and prepare plant foods in a way that give us all the flavor, but none of the addictive properties of meat, dairy, and eggs. Burgers and fries are off the menu, but baked tofu with roasted vegetables and potatoes are on the menu. Spaghetti and meat balls, lasagna, pizza and other Italian dishes will be replaced by McDougall-approved pasta dishes. If you line your baking pan with parchment paper, then you can make an oil-free, vegan pizza. It's delicious, filling, and best of all, it won't damage your health.

If you're going out for dinner, call ahead to the restaurant and ask for simple foods like baked potato, steamed vegetables, salads without dressings, etc. You could bring your own oil-free dressing or sauce to put on your potato and salad. You can also ask the restaurant if they could prepare a simple, oil-free dressing or sauce if they don't allow patrons to bring in their own. The majority of chefs are happy to accommodate dietary preferences.

When eating at home, the best way to approach this plan is to keep it simple in the early days. Boil or bake several potatoes and use them as the base for the next few meals. Baked hash browns for breakfast, potato salad for lunch, potato with steamed vegetables and salsa at dinner; the potato is a versatile vegetable and it will fill you up for hours. Or you can make a large pot of brown rice and use that as your base for meals. Just add an oil-free vegan sauce and some steamed or baked vegetables.

You can purchase frozen spinach and throw that into a pan with onions, carrots, and celery. Add in a ½ to 1 cup of water, cover, and cook over medium high heat for several minutes. Add some hot sauce or cayenne pepper, and a can or two of unsalted black beans. When the beans are heated through, serve over a bed of brown rice or a few potatoes. Another easy and delicious meal made with little fuss or bother.

The other thing is to enlist the support of the people you live with. If you happen to live alone, then it is best you completely clear your fridge and cupboards of all foods derived from animals: beef, chicken, turkey, fish, eggs, and dairy. You also want to get rid of foods that are high in oil, sugar, and salt. For those of you who live with at least one other person, the challenge is to remove from your sight all foods that will tempt you without totally upsetting your spouse or child. Negotiate with them. Ask them to put their snack foods and so on in a place that is off-limits to you. For some people who are very addicted, it may be necessary to put a lock on a cupboard that they don't know the combination to. The reality is some of us need that kind of action if there's any chance for us to get well again. We have to take food addiction seriously.

The animal foods, the meats, the cheeses, and so on, can be the toughest to remove completely from your diet. Talk about a fat bomb, all animal foods are loaded with fats that will clog your arteries and put you at risk of heart disease, cancer, and diabetes.[8] Add to that a spouse who is very unhappy about not being able to eat their usual meat-based meals and you might think it would be World War III!

The thing is, if you truly want to get well and lose your excess weight, you will find a way. In Judith's house, she negotiated with her husband, Dom, to turn their kitchen into a vegan kitchen, but he could still bring home a steak and grill it on the barbecue. This has worked very well for them. Over time, Dom decided to give up dairy, and within weeks his acid reflux cleared up and his diverticulitis went away. He now eats a diet that is roughly 90 percent plant-based. At 63, he takes no medications, which is not the norm for most people his age.[23]

Eighty Percent? One Hundred Percent?

Hopefully, in your kitchen you will be able to achieve a happy compromise for yourself and your family. It's not easy. There are challenges when turning around your diet, and it's usually difficult to follow a new regime 100 percent. If you can do this 80 percent of the time, and you are not suffering with a life-threatening illness, you will most likely have success. Doing this 80 percent means eating a starch-centered, oil-free diet without animal foods at least five and a half days out of seven. Or, to put it differently, you could allow yourself three to four meals per week that are not McDougall-approved, and still see good results with weight loss and improved health.

If you are suffering with heart disease or cancer, however, we would urge you to follow an oil-free, whole food plant-based diet 100 percent. With serious, life-threatening illness, it's best to do this fully without any cheating. Your life is at risk, and we want you to know there are no halfway measures when it becomes a matter of life and death.

The people interviewed in this book independently found out about Dr. John McDougall's starch-centered plan. He has devoted himself to educating the public through his books and various programs. Thanks to Dr. McDougall, we have regained our health and have our lives back. Beginning in chapter five, you are going to meet us and hear our stories. By following Dr. McDougall's dietary program, most of us have lost anywhere from 50 to 100 pounds of excess weight. We have reversed serious, chronic conditions like high blood pressure, high cholesterol, obesity, heart disease, diabetes, and arthritis. *The Starch*

Solution program has certainly improved the quality of our health, and we believe that it has, without a doubt, saved our lives.

Chapter Two
Dr. John McDougall

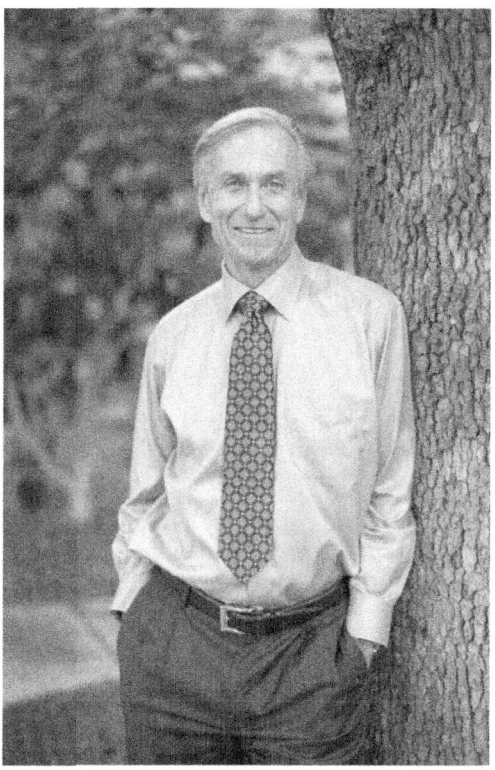

Dr. McDougall is a board-certified internist, in medical practice for over five decades. Thanks to his efforts, the word has spread about the power of a healthy, starch-centerd, plant-based diet to lose weight and get well again. Fifty of us from The Toronto Starch Solution Meetup group gathered to listen to Dr. McDougall talk, in real time, over the internet. This was an important moment for him and us. We are the first group Dr. McDougall has ever encountered that is exclusively dedicated to his Starch Solution program. He was touched and happy to speak with us.

Chapter Two - Dr. John McDougall's Interview

Background and information on Dr. John McDougall

Dr. John McDougall has dedicated his medical career to educating the public on the dangers of eating the Standard American Diet (SAD). He has treated over five thousand patients in person at his McDougall 10-Day Live-In Program at a luxury resort in Santa Rosa, California. He operates this program several times a year and has done so for the past thirty years. During the 10 days, patients lose weight and either reduce or stop their medications. For most of the attendees, it is the first important step they take to recovering from serious illnesses.

There are also hundreds of thousands of people that Dr. McDougall has reached through his many best-selling books, YouTube lectures, interviews, radio and television programs. His website, drmcdougall.com, receives over eight million hits per month. Dr. McDougall also produces a free newsletter that goes out to thirty thousand people each month. It is estimated that one and a half million people have purchased one or more of Dr. McDougall's eleven books.

As well as being a board-certified physician, Dr. McDougall is a researcher. He manages human research trials on the effects of a starch-centered diet to treat disease, and publishes his findings in peer reviewed medical journals. Over the past 40 years, Dr. McDougall has been promoting a whole food, oil-free, plant-based, starch-centered diet, because the diseases he researches are profoundly affected by removing all oils and animal foods from the diet, and eating at least 70% starch.

Dr. McDougall and his wife, Mary McDougall, co-founded Dr. McDougall's Right Foods, which produces prepared plant-based meals for busy people who are looking for quick, healthy meals. They also run a non-profit foundation to raise money for research trials on the benefits of eating a plant-based diet for human health. In addition to their 10-Day Live-In Program, the McDougalls hold 3-Day Programs, Advanced Study weekends, Celebrity Chef weekends, and adventure trips.

Dr. McDougall has played a key role in putting bills before Congress and getting old laws changed. He was instrumental in having Bill SB 380 passed in the state of California, requiring physicians to learn about human nutrition. The reality is that medical doctors have little to no nutritional training. Considering the health benefits of following the kind of diet humans are meant to thrive on, it is very important for physicians to know what kinds of food their patients need to eat to prevent and treat the diseases that are known as the top killers.

Dr. McDougall has co-authored another bill, AB 1478, lobbying for more changes to an outdated medical system. One part of this bill makes it mandatory for doctors to inform their patients that heart surgery will not save their lives in most cases. As shocking as that may sound, that is the unfortunate reality facing most patients. The second piece of this bill also makes it mandatory for doctors to inform their patients that common types of drugs for type 2 diabetes will increase their chances of dying. Considering that surgeries and drugs are being used to manage but not reverse disease, it becomes even more important for the medical establishment to finally recognize that the best chance of survival for the majority of patients is to change their diet.

This interview with Dr. John McDougall was conducted via Skype in November, 2016, with The Toronto Starch Solution Meetup group.

Dr. McDougall, it is wonderful to have you with us here today.

Please tell us about yourself.

I am a doctor, a board-certified internist. I have been in medicine for over 50 years. It has been a very rewarding practice. I have licences to practice medicine in five states. I hold three professorships at three Universities where I teach students. We take medical students and teach them about nutrition and it is now part of their medical training.

I am passionate about reading scientific publications, and I write. I have been trying to spread the word about the power of a healthy diet. It is really an honor to talk to a group that is dedicated to *The Starch Solution*. I don't know of any group that is dedicated to *The Starch Solution*. This is a big deal for me.

Can you tell us why it is so important to eat a starch-centered diet?

Each and every animal has a specific diet. The hippopotamus is designed to eat plants. Horses graze on grasses. My cat Einstein is designed to eat birds and mice. The woodpecker outside my house is designed to eat my house. You know there is a specific diet for each species of animal that they are supposed to eat, to look, feel and function at their best. The question that should be asked by every parent, every scientist and medical doctor is, what is the diet of the human being? There must be one.

Human beings survive on many things. We are very tolerant. We are one of the most resilient of God's creations. We can live on cat food, dog food, dirt food, food you wouldn't feed your animals like licorice and candy bars, and Coca-Cola. It is amazing what the human being can live on. But that is not the question. The question is, what is the ideal diet for the human being?

The human being is a primate, called the greater primate or the greatest primate. The lesser primates like the chimpanzees and the great apes, they are primarily vegetarian. They eat a little bit of meat, a little bit of animal food but they are primarily vegetarians. They live on non-starchy perishable vegetables and fruits.

Based on genetics, humans developed a system that allows us to digest starchy foods efficiently. All the genetic work has been done about how we have more amylase-producing genes that make amylase in order to digest starch, than the other primates. That allowed us two million years ago to develop this unique ability to efficiently digest starch, which is amylose or amylose pectin. That gave us a special opportunity. The great apes and chimpanzees are confined to the equator because that is the only place where you have these perishable non-starchy fruits and vegetables available all year long. Once you leave the equator and go north and south, there are seasons where you don't have food. The primate human developed the ability to digest starches so when they left the equator they had the ability to dig under the ground and find underground storage organs, such as potatoes and sweet potatoes. That enabled them to survive through fall and winter. They were also able to tap into above ground storage organs. These would be legumes and grains, which again last through the winter. Genetically, we evolved from lesser primates into humans and one of the most important DNA genetic changes was our ability to digest starch.

We are starch eaters, always have been. That is why we can live in Toronto, Canada, and Santa Rosa, California because when the fruits and perishable vegetables are gone, we can tap into the source which is starch. If you look back at populations of people, all records of populations show the evidence of us eating starch. I'll give the examples of Mayans and Aztecs who were known as people of the corn. The Incas are the potato eaters in South America. In Asia, the people would often eat rice but they ate many other starches and grains too. The Middle East is known as the bread basket of the world, making breads from grains.

Starch has been the bulk of our calorie intake throughout all of human history, in all populations with rare exceptions. Examples of these rare exceptions are the early Inuit, which really shows how extreme the human being is in terms of the ability to survive in environments that are far from what it was originally designed to live on.

People are opportunistic. They will eat whatever they can get their hands on. Starch is a reliable source of calories. It is easy to get, whereas hunting animals is a tough job. Animals are just not dependable sources of food unless you live in extreme places like Alaska. We are designed as starch eaters but we are survivors too, which is what fools people.

The point is, we are really a tough species. If you want to look at what causes us to look, feel, and function at our best, it is the starch. It is proven by our marathon and triathlon winners. You look at the winners since 1986, 40 percent have been from Kenya, where 80 percent of their diet is primarily corn. Ethiopia, they also have big winners in the endurance events. What you find are real athletes, endurance athletes who live on starch-based diets. Why do they do that? The reason is that athletes win when they eat mostly starches. I also give an example of gladiators from 1800 years ago who have been dug up and had their bones analyzed and they were starch eaters. Gladiators were known as the Barley Men.

People who want to win events, stay alive in the Coliseum, chase their two-year-olds around efficiently, look their best, have the best skin, best body weight, and agility, then starch should be the bulk of their diet. Those who don't live on a starch-based diet are constipated and get all kinds of diseases like rheumatoid arthritis and heart disease and so on. These diseases don't exist in populations that have a diet that is starch-centered.

When I talk to you about populations now, the whole world has become American in terms of eating. In the last 35 years, China has changed from a population where less than one percent of the people had type 2 diabetes, to now, where over 12 percent have type 2 diabetes and half of the population is pre-diabetic. Because of fossil fuels and technology, the majority of people living on planet Earth have McDonald's and Kentucky Fried Chicken in their neighborhoods. They admire the American and Canadian diets. It is hard to see differences in people these days where 35 years ago there were dramatic differences. There were places with a population of tens of millions of people where there was no heart disease, no multiple sclerosis, and there was no rheumatoid arthritis. This was before 1980. After 1980, things changed all over the world.

The most common term used these days is vegan for this kind of diet. We are aspiring to a whole food plant-based diet and I object to all of these terms that are being used because they aren't descriptive enough of what people should be eating. A Mediterranean diet could be made up of chickpeas and eggs. In some people's minds that would be a lacto-ovo-vegetarian. A vegetarian or vegan diet could be made up of coke and potato chips, or at the other extreme kale and broccoli. You could never survive on that.

I know I make a lot of people unhappy because I object to the most common terminology used out there to describe healthier eating. I am also talking about whole food plant-based eating. That is not what you should be calling this. You should be calling this a starch-centered diet because that is the main principle. Starch is the key. For those of you who are listening for the first or the fiftieth time to me, you must understand that starch food is beans and corn, potatoes, sweet potatoes, and rice. We are talking about all the kinds of plant food that have the characteristic of being high in calories respective to other plant foods that are non-starchy and low in calories, like broccoli, cauliflower, kale, lettuce, and celery.

These non-starchy vegetables may add colour, extra vitamins, and minerals to your meal, but you can't live on them. You will starve to death. People try and do it and call it a vegan diet and do it for a day or two, and then say, I can't do it. I can't follow a vegan diet, I am not enjoying this. I can't continue, my stomach is rumbling. There is a very important reason for this. Non-starch vegetables are side dishes at best. If I get to convey to you one important point, it is that you are a starchivore, a starchitarian, a starch-eater. Why? Because that is how you were built.

Going back four million years to hominids, and 750,000 years to homosapiens, the lesser primates go back millions of years before that. The human primate more specifically is built to consume starch. Just like our cat Einstein that is outside on the porch, he is a meat eater. To look, feel, and function at our best, we must live on starch as the central part of our meal.

Once you get this concept, then everything makes sense. You become satisfied and satiated. You will love the food. You get to eat as much as you want. Your bowels start working perfectly. Your cholesterol drops, the type 2 diabetes goes away and the rheumatoid arthritis clears up. All kinds of things happen, but until you get the meat and dairy out of your diet, nothing is going to happen.

In all verifiable history, all human beings have lived on is starch. Let me give you some examples. The easiest ones are people living in Asia. Before 1980, 90 percent of the food consumed in China, Vietnam, and Cambodia was rice. These people were strong, heart-healthy people.

There are some theories out there, like the one on hunter gatherers. The hunter gatherer concept is a true concept in that people are opportunistic. They will eat anything they can get their hands on. Most of what they consumed was gathered. But, the emphasis that goes with the Paleo diet is on the hunting, and the reason for this is something that has been very popular in the United States. It is called sexism.

This is a typical quality of human beings, to be gender biased. Most of the food was not hunted, it was gathered. The hunters were the men. Only a tiny amount of the food was provided by hunting, and it was only sporadic. It wasn't dependable. But because the hunters were the men, that is where all the glory and the talk centered around, and it still does today. The talk is of how important hunting was in terms of consuming food for your people. It is simply not true. Most of the food was provided by the gatherers but they were the underclass. They had sexism in their society. The men were the ones who got all the glory.

The diet I recommend is based on starch with the addition of fruits and vegetables. I don't recommend that people eat any meat or any oil. When you read my new book, *The Healthiest Diet on the Planet*, you will see that it clearly teaches you that there are two categories of food poisoning. One category of food poisoning is animal food: frogs and snakes and whales and cows and pigs and birds and so on. The other category of food poisoning is oil: like olive oil, corn oil, safflower oil and so on.

Well, when I say that to most groups, not necessarily this group, they say there is nothing left to eat. I just told you, your diet is primarily supposed to be starch. That is what *The Starch Solution* teaches and that is what you are learning in this class. If you read *The Healthiest Diet on the Planet*, then that is what you will learn, that is what you will start to put into everyday life.

I told you about Einstein my cat a few minutes ago. My cat, he is a carnivore. He eats meat and likes meat. If I took him to the grocery store and walked him down the meat aisle, he'd be right over top of the counter and chewing that meat up like his life depended on it, but that is his food. When I walk down the meat aisle at Safeway or any other grocery store, just the sight and smell of meat makes me nauseated. It is disgusting. Just think about it when you are in the meat aisle. It is really foul because it is not your food.

Now, let's take Einstein. Let's say I decide that I am going to change Einstein's diet because I am an ethical vegetarian. I am not going to give Einstein any more meat. I am going to give Einstein baked potatoes because that is the McDougall diet. Potatoes are a big part of the diet. So, what I do is, I bring Einstein in the house and throw a baked potato down in front of him. What do you think Einstein is going to do with that potato? Maybe bat it around a little bit, but he is not going to eat it, because that is not his food. Einstein will be starving to death because I am throwing potatoes at him three times a day and he is still not eating them.

So, what I decided to do in the cause of science and maybe to keep Einstein alive, I am going to mash those potatoes and put them in his stomach in a gastric tube. I am just going to pump those mashed potatoes into his stomach. Well, what happens? Two weeks later Einstein is almost dead. He is withering. I'm losing my cat.

Well, then I think about what I should do. As your doctors were taught and I was taught, the way you make people healthy is you exercise them or you help them relieve their stress, so I am going to apply that to Einstein. I am going to take out the old dog leash and run Einstein around the block a couple of times a day. What do you think is going to happen to Einstein after that heavy exercise regime? He is still dying, almost dead.

I decide the next thing I am going to do is deal with the stress and psychological issues. I am going to reach down four or five times a day and rub Einstein's ears and give him a nice pet. What do you think is going to happen to Einstein with that therapy? He'll soon be dead, that's what will happen. You see, the only way I am going to get Einstein well, is to put him back on the food that he is designed for.

It is the same thing with you. You go to the doctor. You are sick. You are overweight. You have diabetes. You have high blood pressure. You are constipated. You have digestive issues. You have inflammatory arthritis. You have multiple sclerosis, on and on and on. What the doctor does, instead of treating the cause of the problem, the doctor gives you a bunch of pills and tells you to go see the psychologist and get more exercise. But, until you understand the cause of your problems, you will stay fat and sick. It is the food. Until you understand you are a starch eater, until you fulfill your design, you are never going to get well. I don't care how many pills they throw at you for these chronic diseases. I don't care how many psychiatrists or psychologists you visit. I don't care if you become a triathlon runner, you will continue to stay sick until you change your food. You may get thinner by exercising but you are still going to be sick. That is the basis of the way I prevent disease. I have people get on a healthy diet. The way I cure chronic diseases, is to take people and put them back on the human diet they are designed to eat which is a starch-based diet.

Dr. McDougall, what kinds of food should we be eating then?

A starch-based diet is what you should be eating. Starch eating is the basis of the human diet. I just want to tell you what to eat, even though there is a picture of pancakes on the cover of my book. For breakfast, eat whole grain cereals like oats. You can also enjoy waffles and French toast, which we have recipes for. We have well over 3000 recipes published. We have a mobile McDougall cookbook app that has 1000 recipes in it and is available on my website.

For lunch, you can think about things like: pea soup, bean soup, lentil soup, tomato soup. These are soups you already love. You just leave the oil and the meat out and they taste just as good, in fact, they taste better to me.

For dinner, you can have bean burritos, spaghetti in marinara sauce, vegetables over rice. When you think back to your childhood, your grandparents lived on these kinds of food, particularly if they were from non-North American countries. If you have relatives from countries like China, Japan, and so on, you realize that your parents and grandparents lived well and loved the food they made. I want to make sure you all understand this is not about sacrifice. This is the best tasting food that there is. It accomplishes great health, and saves the environment.

Did you know that the environmental impact of beef is 100 times greater than that of potatoes? We are interested in saving the world for you, your children and your grand kids. I am talking about a diet that is in every way right for you. It will fix your health. It will fix the environment and it will take care of medical costs. It will save the cruelty of killing a billion animals a day to feed people worldwide. Because it is true and right, it must be right in every aspect. That is why it is important that you understand the full implication of this way of eating. You get to eat as much as you want. It is right in every single way that you look at it.

The crazy thing is that people think we are deprived eating this way, or that we don't enjoy what we eat. Last night, Mary made a bean stew over purple sweet potatoes and it was amazing.

Dr. McDougall, people are taught and believe that meat and dairy are health foods and are a necessary and essential part of a healthy diet. Is this true?

Well at first, we must discuss why people believe this. The reason people believe we have to eat meat and dairy and fish and poultry is because of marketing. Marketing is something that every business does. It will find something unique about this product and position it in the public's eye as necessary. It is called unique positioning. The meat and dairy and egg industries, they have been doing this for at least a hundred years. They have taken something unique about their product and told the public that this is the most important nutrient. For example, if I say calcium, you will say milk. Or, if I say protein, you will say meat. If I say omega-3 fats, you will say fish.

The truth of the matter is there has never in all of human history, in all the scientific research, been a case of calcium deficiency on a natural diet. It has never occurred. There has never been a case of protein deficiency on any natural diet. Omega-3 fats cannot be made by animals, including fish. They are only made by plants. But, this is just business. People shouldn't think about this as a conspiracy. This is just normal business and we have been taught the most important nutrients are calcium, protein, and omega-3 fats. These deficiencies don't exist and plants always supplied all the protein, calcium, and omega-3 fats that we need.

When you eat a starch-based diet with fruits and vegetables, it is the most nutrient rich diet of them all. But for advertising reasons, people don't focus on vitamin C and beta carotene, or plant formed vitamin E and the other phyto-nutrients. It is just part of the marketing scheme.

Why is it important that we stop eating meat, dairy, and all animal products?

First, animal foods completely lack basic nutrients like vitamin C and dietary fibre. They lack beta carotene. They are nutritionally deficient. A cat doesn't need vitamin C because it makes it itself. That is the way its system is. For us humans, we don't make ascorbic acid (vitamin C), so we must take it in with our food, which is only found in plants. Beta carotene is only found in plants.

The other thing is these animal foods are overloaded with nutrients that place a serious burden on the body. For example, the protein found in animal foods is so much more protein than we need. We only need five percent of our calories from protein. Well, meat may be 30 percent protein, turkey may be 60 to 80 percent protein. When we eat these animal foods we take in a lot of substances that our body must deal with, and it places a serious burden on our body. For example, the protein places a burden on the bones because it is acidic. The bones dissolve and we develop osteoporosis, and when the bone material is excreted out of the body, it collects in the kidneys and calcifies and causes kidney stones. Our bodies must deal with an extra burden of protein.

We must deal with the burden of fat. Fat is the metabolic dollar for when food isn't available, so eating animals is a burden in terms of fat. Some animals are low-fat. If they are low-fat, they are very high in protein and you can develop serious problems with low-fat animal foods. Most animals have a lot of fat in them and that fat you eat is the fat you wear. You can develop obesity.

Animals today are even more special in terms of their burden. They are hyper accumulators of environmental chemicals. The environmental chemicals such as DDT and PCB are chemicals that are used worldwide. Many other chemicals are produced as side products from manufacturing. These environmental chemicals get into the food chain and what happens is they get magnified. They bio-accumulate. The chemicals end up in grasses and grains, and then are eaten by the cow.

They increase in concentration. It was after World War II, when environmental chemicals became so prevalent. It is such a serious problem today. If you look at the Inuit and check their body tissues, you find their mammalian milk, their breast milk, and their other body tissues are so toxic with environmental poisons that they are considered waste hazards. For example, the breast milk of an Inuit woman has ten times more environmental contaminants than a woman in southern Canada. By eating these animals, you end up taking in poisons that give you illnesses like cancer and brain damage.

The other thing is that animals are the source of microbe food poisoning. We hear all the time about outbreaks of listeria on cantaloupes. We heard one in Europe three or four years ago about how the cantaloupes contained listeria. Listeria is a bacterium that can cause serious illness and death. Tomatoes that are contaminated with salmonella or e-coli were in the news recently. The apples out in Seattle at one of the apple companies almost went out of business because of the e-coli in their apple products.

What people need to realize is that plants don't grow any of these organisms. The only reason these organisms are present is because of animal excrement. A cow walks through the apple field and poops on the ground, then the apple falls on the ground and that is how that apple delivers e-coli. The apple never developed e-coli. It came from animal waste.

You see that a lot these days in the food processing industry. Half of the chicken flock are seriously contaminated with Staphylococcus aureus. They call it chicken fecal soup. The animal foods provide food poisoning in the form of chemicals and bacteria and viruses like bovine leukemia virus, bovine immunodeficiency virus, and other cancer viruses, prions like mad cow, and parasites like trichinella. There are hundreds of thousands, if not millions of cases of food poisoning every year in the US and Canada from these bacteria. The source is not the vegetables. The source is the animal foods.

Meat and dairy have inadequate and improper nutrients for us humans. They're overloaded with fat and protein, and totally deficient of carbohydrates, which is the fuel the human body burns. The primary source of energy is glucose. Animal food contains no glucose at all unless you are looking at cow's milk, and that is still loaded with chemicals and microbes.

The other reason is that it is cruel to kill a billion animals a day to eat. Once you become aware, it is unbelievable and unacceptable that billions of animals a year are brutally killed here in the US for food that we not only don't need, but is making us sick. Billions of animals are slaughtered every year worldwide. The way this business is run, it is cruel by anybody's standard. I don't know anyone who goes to a slaughterhouse or processing plant and isn't repulsed by what is going on. I know even hard core meat eaters, when they walk down the aisle of a supermarket and they go through the meat section, the sights and smells leave them nauseated.

The real problem is the environment. There was an article in our paper this morning that there are hundreds of villages in Alaska that are being flooded and are being destroyed because of rising levels of sea water. The storms and the droughts, and all the other things that are going on are due to manmade pollution. California just passed a law in the last few days that puts a cap on the amount of cow flatulence that can be allowed in California's environment. Livestock accounts for half of the greenhouse gases in the world.

We are in a situation where the environmental impact of livestock is serious. Mother Nature doesn't give a damn. The question is when and how soon will it happen. From what I have seen, over the last ten years, we are not talking about a hundred years from now. We are talking about a massive threat to the planet, and it is going to occur to the point where our very survival will be threatened within the next 20 years.

Let's be optimistic for a minute. Let's say the world leaders got up today and told the world from this point on, we are not consuming chicken, beef, pork and fish or we will put you in jail, like we would a heroin addict, if you raise or eat them. Our world leaders could make it a law tomorrow. In fact, we probably need to kill off all of the animals being raised for food. If we did that, I wonder what would be the consequences. Let's just say we stopped this tomorrow and we took our armies out of the Middle East, out of Iraq and Iran. We fought every forest fire we could and stopped all the forest fires that are contributing to the world greenhouse gases. Our soldiers were out there planting crops, and we put every effort we possibly could into turning this around. It might give us enough time, but it must be done right now. This is an emergency. With all the other things that are being promoted such as electric cars and solar energy, if it was a worldwide effort, a greater effort than we put into World War II, then maybe we could save ourselves and prevent total extinction.

Dr. McDougall, we have several people here who are vegetarians and they are wondering why no oil? Why is that so important?

I'll tell you why, oil is a poison. It is the second category of poison. Oil is not food. Oil is an isolated extract that comes from various foods like corn, olives, safflower, and primrose. They take and they extract one ingredient and leave everything else behind. When you eat oil in its natural form, like in an orange, or a potato, or rice, then of course, oil is very safe and it has all the proteins, vitamins, minerals, phytochemicals and so on that are necessary to properly digest it. But when you strip the oil out of a food, what you end up with is not a food. You end up with a substance that at best can act like a medication, and at worst is a poison.

Let me tell you how these oils affect you. When you eat it, the destiny of this oil is to go into your body fat. If you eat corn oil, you will be full of corn oil. Let me put it this way. If I came up to you with a needle and I stuck it into your buttocks, thigh, or abdomen and sucked out the fat and took it to the lab, I can tell you what you like to eat. If your body fat was full of trans fats then I know you like margarines and shortenings. If your body fat was full of omega-3 fats, I would guess you were into fish or flaxseed or flaxseed oils. In other words, the fat you eat is the fat you wear.

The first thing to understand about oil is it has the highest calorie concentration of any food. It is nine calories per gram. It is easily transferred from your fork and spoon to your butt and your thighs. It is the primary cause of being overweight. Not eating oil is one of the most important things to do if you want to lose weight. The objective is to get the oil out of the food, and to add a note, that means the nuts and seeds and avocados too. Isolated oil is immediately deposited in your body fat and in your skin, and causes greasy hair and greasy skin, which contributes to acne.

Oil also has pharmacological properties. Omega-3 fats thin the blood.

That may be good if you are trying to prevent a heart attack which occurs because of a blood clot. But, what happens if you get into an auto accident? You are more likely to bleed to death. The Inuit, who eat a lot of omega-3s, are known for fatal nose bleeds. This oil also suppresses the immune system. That may be good if you have rheumatoid arthritis because it acts like an aspirin and suppresses the immune system, but it suppresses the whole immune system, so as a result, cancer grows much faster.

There are experiments done on animals showing that tumour growth is a thousand times greater when they feed flaxseed oil to the experimental animal, the rat in this case, rather than having them on a low-fat diet. Oil also suppresses the immune system when you want to avoid getting infections. When you suppress the immune system, you are more likely to get viral and bacterial infections.

Oil is toxic. It is not food. It is one of the most important things for you to get away from if you are trying to lose weight and trying to avoid cancer. I was mentioning the omega-3 fats, but there are the omega-6 fats that come from safflower and corn. The omega-6 fats, when they studied them in opposition to animal fats, were found to be more toxic to the arteries, causing more death and more disease than even lard and animal fat. These things need to be removed from your diet.

Dr. McDougall, what is your opinion of ground flaxseeds?

I think you are damaging the flaxseed. You make whatever is in it more potent. The good thing about the components of flaxseed is omega-3 oil, which is what flaxseed is promoted for. When you grind it up, the omega-3 becomes more available, which means you thin the blood more and you suppress the immune system more, and you are going to get more fat than if you eat the whole flaxseed. You don't improve the quality of the food be it a vegetable or a fruit by hitting it 10,000 times with a steal blade.

Dr. McDougall, how does your eating approach affect inflammation?

Go to my January 2011 Newsletter, or read my new book *The Healthiest Diet on the Planet*. They discuss inflammation and show you all of the scientific research. By the way, the January 2011 Newsletter was dedicated to the books, *Grain Brain and Wheat Belly* which are smoke and mirrors.

My newsletter does look at different types of food and their various effects on inflammation, as determined by inflammatory markers like C-reactive protein. What is found consistently is that animal foods create inflammation, tremendous inflammation in fact, and vegetable foods including wheat and various grains suppress inflammation.

The common story out there about the Paleo diet and the hunter gatherer, is that we were hunters. Well, it is just nonsense. The idea that eating animal food is good for inflammation is not true. That is not what the scientific research says. The scientific research says the exact opposite, eating animal food causes inflammation. I presented that information in my January 2011 Newsletter and also in my new book. Go look up the studies. If you want to see the science and your friends say otherwise and they tell you that wheat causes inflammation or grain causes inflammation, you say, "Well excuse me, let's take a look at the basic research that comes out of The National Academy of Science, and The American Journal of Nutrition, and ask them where do they get their ideas about this."

People buy into the wrong information because people love to hear good news about their bad habits. We have been raised on diets of pepperoni pizza and hot dogs and now we have the All-American Burger, and Kentucky Fried Chicken. The All-American Burger combines a hot dog, hamburger, bacon, and cheese all together in one sandwich. When you can eat something like that any time you like, then you know why people love to hear good news about their bad habits.

Dr. McDougall, has your message changed at all in forty years?

No, my message hasn't changed. That is the thing that they will say to me, in fact. My son is a medical doctor in Portland, Oregon. He finally got around to reading my New York Times bestselling book, *The McDougall Plan*. He started out with *The Starch Solution* and he said to me, "Why did you write another book? You said it all in *The McDougall Plan* which you published about 35 years ago."

He is right. I've said the same thing in that book that I say in the new book, *The Healthiest Diet on the Planet*. It is just that the method of communication has improved greatly. My ability to communicate the message and make it more palatable and understandable to everybody from the top scientists in the world to somebody who has a fifth grade education is what has changed over the years.

We have had 13 national bestselling books. Seven of them are still in print. No, my message hasn't changed because the truth doesn't change.

Dr. McDougall, why is obesity on the rise?

It is on the rise. Thirty-eight percent of the population of the United States and Canada is obese. Medical doctors had been told that we have to put a cap on this, because the obesity rate has escalated to over 34 percent in the last couple of years, and then this year they reported that the obesity rate is 38 percent. Aside from obesity, overweight is approaching 80 percent of the population in the US and Canada.

Back in 1980, 35 years ago, there was no obesity in China. Obesity in India was confined to the very upper tier, the very upper class of people. In 35 years, that has changed. Now, they report in India that it is not just the upper class, it is the middle class that suffers from type 2 diabetes and obesity the same as the upper class does.

In China, they just published a paper where they said before 1980, there was less than one percent of the population with type 2 diabetes. As of the year 2013, 12 percent of the Chinese population suffers from diabetes. There is a tremendous rise of obesity in countries that were less rich five years ago, but now they have become rich or richer than Americans, like China, for example. They will soon have the same obesity rate as we do.

Let's get back to the US and Canada. When I was growing up, my mom fixed a diet for us that she thought was proper. She thought it would give you enough calcium and protein, which are the two messages of the meat and dairy industry broadcasted because that is their unique marketing proposition. I'll remind you again that there has never been a case of calcium or protein deficiency ever recorded in the world literature on any natural diet. However, it was decided to teach my mom that of all the nutrients, it was calcium and protein that were most important, and that came from industry. My mom served us eggs for breakfast and at dinner, we had chicken. Sometimes we had ham and steak and so on. We were eating the typical Western diet, except for one thing, my mom had to fix the food, and it was only available three times a day.

Nowadays, it is the accessibility of the food. Our calorie intake has increased tenfold and that is brought up in *The Healthiest Diet on the Planet*. Our calorie intake has increased over a thousand calories per person per day from the time that I was a child until now. Now, how is that possible? What happened? Well, it is because of the tremendous amount of advertising that had taken place, plus the convenience.

Today, to get your food, all you have to do is drive along the road, take a side turn into a driveway, roll down your window and it appears. Then, you roll up your window and drive another mile or two and take another turn into a driveway, roll down your window and the food appears again.

It is the accessibility. Plus, the food industry has dedicated a tremendous amount of money to in-house research, to produce the most palatable food possible. They make the food addictive, and that's their goal. The book, *Sugar, Fat and Salt* by Michael Moss, goes into how industry has scientific departments dedicated to making their food irresistible to you. The food is subsidized and cheap. Unless you know the truth, people think they are getting a bargain at a fast food restaurant.

Dr. McDougall, can the McDougall diet help someone with Crohn's disease who has had part of their intestine surgically removed?

The Starch Solution can help tremendously. Crohn's disease is a disease of The Western diet. It did not exist prior to 1980. We have many Star McDougallers on the website that had ulcerative colitis. They changed their diet and cured their disease.

Now, to the person who is asking this question, I know you have had a lot of damage to your intestinal tract and you have had surgery and those kinds of permanent changes. They may leave you with residual problems but I bet, and you can write me an email and tell me I am wrong, but I bet, if you follow the starch-based diet, no oils, no animals, lots of starch, where 70 to 90 percent of your diet is starch, I would bet that you will see improvement by the end of the week. Within four months, you'll say to yourself, I cannot believe that I missed this and I am angry that I missed this, why didn't my doctor teach me this?

With regards to nutrition and cancer, and hearing that several cancers are related directly to nutrition, is that true with any cancer? What about lung cancer specifically?

There are cancers caused by other things other than food, like radiation and arsenic. With lung cancer, this discussion starts in my February 2015 Newsletter and my July 2016 Newsletter. If you are interested, look up on the search engine a doctor named Ernst Wynder. He was one of my friends and one of my mentors from many years ago. I met him in 1978. He was the head of the American Health Foundation, which was a group of 200 scientists that started The Journal of Preventative Medicine and published over 800 papers. He was one of the world experts on cancer.

We had breakfast together in 1978, at the first diet and cancer conference. I initiated the conversation because I wanted to get to know this man. He said, "John, I am the one that discovered the connection and made it public between cigarette smoking and tobacco." He published his first article in JAMA in 1950. He said to me, "I went to the cancer experts and said to them, 'Smoking cigarettes causes lung cancer,' and they said, 'Naw, how could that be?'" And then Wynder said, "I told them, 'You take this tube of tobacco and you light it and you suck the smoke into your lungs and it causes lung cancer.' They couldn't believe it. After ten years, I went back to the same people and I said to them, 'Eating meat causes colon cancer,' and they said, 'Naw, how could that be?' I said, 'You chew the stuff up and swallow it and it gets into your colon and causes colon cancer.'" Dr. Wynder published many, many articles on the kind of diet that was causing colon cancer.

Regarding your question about diet and lung cancer, diet has a huge influence on lung cancer. One example is the Japanese in the 1950s. At that time, 60 percent of the males in Japan smoked cigarettes. When they compared them to cigarette smokers in the US, they found that in

Japan they had one quarter of the incidence of lung cancer. Their diet was mainly a starch-based diet. The reason is you inhale this toxic substance from the cigarette. If you have a healthy body, you are better able to defend and repair the damage from the tobacco and associated combustion products. What you eat has a tremendous effect on lung cancer, the kind caused by tobacco.

There is another kind of lung cancer that we see in non-smokers, adenocarcinoma. It is not related to smoking, it is related to diet and therefore can be prevented with the right diet. However, non-dietary cancers due to irritation from tobacco respond to an improved diet. You get the same results with skin cancer, when people have precancerous lesions, or squamous or basal cell carcinomas. In the New England Journal of Medicine, a study was published showing if patients eat a low-fat diet, they will have two to six times fewer occurrences.

In my November 2015 newsletter, I wrote about the effect of diet on the people who have cancer: colon, breast, prostate and melanoma. The reason I wrote this newsletter is the American Cancer Society came out in February 2015 and made it official to the public that people who have cancer need to change their diet. They will live longer even after they have cancer. This is now an official announcement.

Dr. McDougall, two-thirds of the population are overweight and most people believe carbohydrates and starches make you fat. Your starch-centered program seems to help people get thin almost effortlessly. How?

Starch is the food for human beings. Its primary element and energy source is sugar and our bodies and cells run on sugar. In fact, some of the cells of the body only run on sugar. They can't burn protein or fat. If you don't have any sugar in your diet in the form of carbohydrates, then the body must convert protein into sugar to keep the kidney and red bloods cells alive. It is the right food for the body. If you take in more carbohydrates than you need, then the body will convert a little bit of it into fat, however, it's not much fat. The body is not very good at doing that. Therefore, it is just the right food for people in terms of keeping them healthy, trim, and strong. Those are the people that win the marathons and triathlons, as we have already talked about.

Fats are the metabolic dollars that are stored in the body. Fat is just moved from the fork and right into the digestive tract to the blood vessels, and gets shunted into the fat cells. When you get the fat out of the diet, the fat will stop being stored. When you replace it with carbohydrates, it is difficult for carbohydrates to be converted to fat. That is why every population that is starch-based doesn't have fat people.

When I was a young man, I was peripherally involved in the Vietnam War. We would watch videos of people from Vietnam and Cambodia. I would see a gathering of 100,000 people and there was not one fat person. Today, in those countries, there are many fat people, specifically business people and politicians and so on. Think of the leader of North Korea. He didn't get that way eating rice. The reason that you stay trim on a starch-based diet is that it's the diet for people.

Dr. McDougall, a common challenge seems to be cravings for salt, sugar and oil, and how that seems to be the daily battle field for a lot of people. Do you have any helpful hints? Is it just willpower?

We are naturally attracted to salt and sugar, because that is what we are supposed to eat. It shouldn't be something that you have to fight. We have seven taste buds. We have salt and sugar on the tip of the tongue which causes you to seek sugar because that is what you are supposed to use for fuel. That sugar would be things like fruit, corn and potatoes. We have the salt taste bud because we need minerals so we naturally seek salt. We have two taste buds that detect poisonous and medicinal tastes, which is the sour and bitter toward the back of the tongue.

The fifth taste bud is umami, identified by a Japanese scientist named Kikunae Ikeda in the early 1900s. It is a taste for monosodium glutamate. That is the one that they say attracts us to meat, but that is not true. That is mostly stimulated by MSG.

There is a sixth taste bud that was recently discovered about 10 years ago for fat, but it is a taste bud of repulsion not attraction. People who can taste fat don't eat it. People who can't taste it don't have that as a dominant taste bud. They eat a lot more fat and are more likely to be obese.

About six months ago Oregon State University published a very important paper on the seventh taste bud and that was the taste bud for starch. What they did was they blocked the sweet tasting taste buds on the tip of the tongue and then they fed people various foods so the sweet tasting taste buds were blocked up. They found that they had extremely strong attraction to starch foods like bread and rice. That taste bud was identified as strong as our attraction to sweet. Research discovering a starch tasting taste bud is crucial. I would say that the body is working as it should be. It is properly being attracted to starch, sweet, and salt.

The problem is that industry knows this. They don't know the starch part that was just recently discovered, but they do know the sugar and salt part, so that is how they sell you their products. They make foods that the customer buys, and they have scientific teams in these food companies that spend all their days trying to make their products as attractive and irresistible as possible.

We are not attracted to fat, and oil is disgusting. We identify a bad restaurant as a greasy spoon. When people get fat and oils on their hands they immediately wash with soap. They are repulsed by fat, and they also get a strong detergent out to clean off the grease that ends up on their kitchen stoves.

So why is fat in the food? People say it gives you a smooth taste and texture to the food. I don't know if that is very important. The reason they add oil to fast foods is it allows the things that we like to be incorporated into the foods more efficiently. Oil allows the salt to stick to the potato chips and French fries. Oil allows sugar to attach to the donuts. Have you ever tried a fried donut with no sugar, which I did in my childhood? It's just a greasy blob. It's a way to get the sugar to stick. It is the same thing with herbs and spices. The way you get herbs and spices to stick to salad leaves is you use oil. It is an adherent. That is why oil is in the food. It allows the things that you like to easily attach to your food.

Dr. McDougall, is the reason we lose weight on your program due to removing the oil in our diet?

Yes, fat is the main thing. I have a slogan that I ask people to repeat in their head as a reminder. A mantra they say all day long, "The fat you eat is the fat you wear." When you stop eating the fat, then you stop accumulating it. When you start eating carbohydrates instead of fat, you become more active. The body naturally wants to be trim and strong to survive. This is a basic natural survival instinct. When you stop eating the fat, and you have 50 or 60 pounds of extra fat on, the body says, now I can finally get rid of this. You were force feeding me fat at such great levels I could do nothing but store it. Now that it has a chance to re-regulate and burn the carbohydrates, it naturally burns off the fat. This is all natural.

There are probably more detailed chemical explanations that can be given to you but it is just the fact that looking like a butterball is not what a human being is supposed to look like. When you stop the fat, you stop that unnatural, anti-survival appearance, because you can't run away from a sabre-toothed tiger. You can't get into the cave which has a small entrance if you are too fat. One of the natural tendencies of any species is for it to survive. Survival is an inborn trait that every species has, from a mosquito to an elephant. Once you take it out of an abnormal environment, which is anti-survival, it will do everything it can to re-adapt so it can do its primary thing which is to survive.

Dr. McDougall, people often talk about eating only lean meats and avoiding carbohydrates. What do you think of that type of diet?

A diet that only allows lean meats is called rapid starvation, where 35 percent or more of the calories are made from protein. Explorers back in the old days would live on these lean animal diets and they would die from rapid starvation from all that protein. For the Inuit, their primary calorie source is not protein, it is the fat that is in the seal and the walrus. You can only go so high in terms of protein before you go into rapid starvation, but there is a lot of fat in meats.

Dr. Caldwell Esselstyn recently came out with a statement, "Medicine is on the verge of a seismic revolution in health." Do you agree with that statement?

I don't know what he means by that statement. I don't see the drug companies being stopped. In my next newsletter, you will see a report that says that in August of this year, we have spent more money on hospitals, medicines, and other standard medical therapies than ever in all of history since 1984. Drug companies are the most profitable of all companies. Their business is growing leaps and bounds over any other company. I don't see change. If Dr. Esselstyn is saying that that the world is going to change because we are on some precipice of change, I have got to talk to him. He is a good friend.

I do, however, believe that change is coming. It won't be stopped. But it has nothing to do with the will of human beings. It has to do with the growth of our human population and the environmental changes that are occurring as the consequences of global warming.

Do you think we are still a long way away from a starch-centered diet taking hold and becoming the norm?

We are changing. The planet is changing with the efforts we are all making. People like yourself are changing. There are more vegetarians and more vegans; more people that understand starches are good food. It is changing. But the question is, is it changing fast enough? My answer is not as I see it. But, something tremendous could come out.

When you read my newsletter, you'll see a video of Barack Obama and Michelle Obama who, by the way, live on a starch-based diet. Michelle declares herself vegan, and I know for many reasons that Barack eats like we do. For one, he was one of my students when he was 15 years old, so he learned all this. He was in my class. I didn't know who Barry was, except that he was the only black kid in Kuno High School. We had many conversations after my lectures. He knows this. He has been in office eight years and it is not entirely his fault. The Republicans have done everything they can to stop everything he wanted to do.

Bill Clinton started following our diet, and I do take some credit for it. We have Bill Clinton, our 42nd president, Barack Obama, our 44th president, and Dennis Kucinich, who is our Ohio Representative, Hawaiian senator Mike Gabbard, all vegan, all trying to push for healthy diets in the nation and in schools.

Dr. McDougall, if you were not a healthcare practitioner, just an ordinary person like us, what would you do to promote this way of eating?

Nathan Pritikin was one of my heroes. He was an engineer, not a doctor. He was one of my greatest influences. I have many mentors in my life. He had the greatest influence on me of any doctor or non-doctor in the world. He was just an ordinary person. Maybe I would have been just as effective as being a non-doctor. I don't think that being a doctor or a scientist, or having credentials is crucial. I think you just need to be a good communicator and remain strong in your beliefs.

My wife Mary is 70 years old, and she is a beautiful woman. We were in Whole Foods yesterday and a woman in her forties just walked up to Mary and said, "You are such a beautiful woman." I said, "Fortunately she has been my wife for 45 years." In some ways, just looking good conveys a message.

Whatever your skills and personality, you can communicate the truth to people. You don't have to be a doctor or a dietitian. You don't have to be a billionaire. Some of these things may help, but in many ways, all of us can be important. For example, my hairstylist has a sign on the back of her car that says, "If you want to become a vegan in four and a half hours, watch *Forks Over Knives*, *Cowspiracy*, and *Earthlings*." It is actually plastered over the whole back window of her car. As far as other things, to get people to eat right I think you can appeal to people's religious teachings as well. The Bible clearly states that we aren't supposed to eat very much meat.

People ask me, "How do I get my ten-year-old to eat this way?" I say to them, take them to the farm yard to pet a cow or a pig and make them realize that this is what they are eating. People don't say they are eating a pig chop. I'm not saying I'm eating a cow butt. Let's call it what it is. You can appeal to their common sense. Walk them down the meat aisle and tell them to take a big sniff. Bring your cat along with you and see what your cat does. Say to them, "You can have all the beef and chicken you want, but you can't cook it. Okay, I'll let you cook it but you can only boil it and then you can eat it. You can't put anything on it to cover up the flavor."

There are different ways to appeal to people. Another way is to make it really positive. Show them how good the food really is. People think we are suffering. Boy, I'll tell you, tonight we are having mashed potatoes, and creamy gravy, and a package of frozen corn boiled. I combine those in a bowl and add a little salt and pepper to taste. That is my favourite meal of all. With Mary's creamy gravy, you could eat cardboard and it would taste good.

Dr. McDougall, over the years, what have been some of the most memorable healings that you have witnessed with *The Starch Solution* **program?**

That is a relative thing. I have seen people lose weight. I have seen people lose 60 pounds, 100 pounds, 120 pounds, purposefully. I have seen people get rid of constipation, which is miraculous. I have seen cancers cured. I don't have a particular study, but I do have many studies from my February 2000 newsletter of how people who eat well survive longer. I have seen people with bodies full of cancers that have disappeared. I don't know how often that occurs. I have seen many, many cases of heart disease reversed. It is kind of relative. If you are a person who has a bowel movement every twelve days, this diet is a miracle. If you have arthritis and you can't get out of your chair and now you can walk, that is a miracle.

I really can't say what would be the most miraculous thing I've seen. The assessment of that miracle lies in the eyes of the beholder, the person who gains the benefits. I have never seen anyone who is suffering from The Western diet not get better. Sometimes they are left with residual disease and scars, like somebody who had arthritis in their hip and had to have a hip replacement. The hip doesn't grow back. Everybody gets dramatically better when they get off The Western diet and switch to starches. We are all miracles.

I want to close by saying one thing about Canadians as opposed to Americans. You have a Canadian Services Task Force that helps you prevent cancers. We have the United States Preventative Services Task Force. I want you to know, last year, the Canadian Task Force told Canadians to stop getting colonoscopies for screening. Yes, you folks did. The US Preventative Task Force still supports the colonoscopy industry, but they admit there has never been a randomized control trial that shows colon cancer and related mortality.

There is no data that shows any screening technique, whether we're talking about mammography, breast self examination, rectal examination, colonoscopy, or fecal blood test, that shows that any of these tests ever improve overall mortality. They just determine how you are going to die. They don't extend your life. If they find a colon polyp and it is large and pre-malignant, they remove it. You have less chance of dying of colon cancer but in the process of discovering this polyp, they end up killing an equal number of people as you end up saving. So, overall mortality is not changed. These screening techniques are widely promoted in the US and Canada. In fact, no European country has ever promoted colonoscopy for screening. Canada used to, up until just a few months ago. The US still does. They are still tied into the multibillion-dollar colonoscopy business.

In conclusion, what I want to ask you is to help save the world. The world is worth saving by eating a starch-based diet. You just never know. My grandkids will never look back and say, "Grandpa, why didn't you try harder?" Grandpa works 14 hours a day to turn this thing around. My whole family eats this way. It is just a matter of opening your eyes. Let's save the world. We are in this together.

Chapter Three

McDougall's McFacts
What We Have Learned
From Dr. McDougall

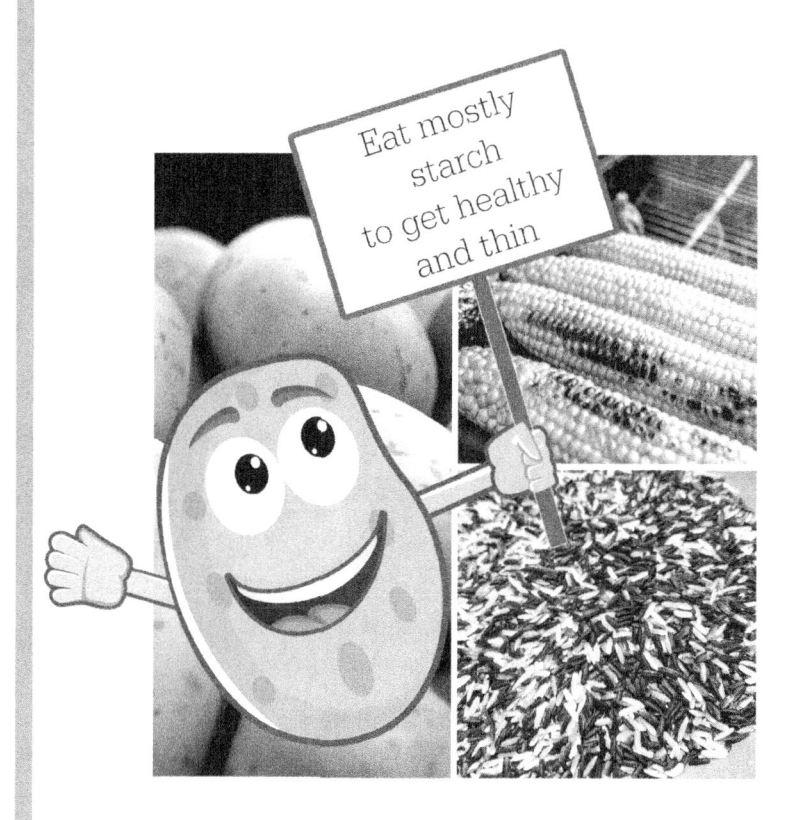

Chapter Three - McDougall's McFACTS

What We Have Learned from Dr. John McDougall

What is a "McFact"?

In this chapter, we are presenting a summation of many points about healthy and unhealthy living, the science of nutrition, and about developing a healthy lifestyle that Dr. McDougall has emphasized over his 40-year career. We use the term "McFact" as a term of endearment and as a Dr. John McDougall approved scientific statistic. These facts are based on scientific research but are not necessarily embraced by the general public or medical establishment as of yet.

The Best Diet of All

McFact: *The Starch Solution* **diet prevents most disease.**
People who indulge in the standard Western diet, loaded in dairy products like milk, cheese and yogurt, meats, fish, eggs and processed junk food, will most likely shorten their lives. They will be prone to getting sick and fat, and suffer with chronic degenerative diseases. These diseases are often preventable by eating a starch-centered diet with added fruits and vegetables.[1,2]

McFact: Your body has the ability to heal itself with the right

food.

Your body has an innate ability to heal itself, if you give it the right food, which is a starch-centered diet. Plants have an abundant amount of 11 of the 13 essential nutrients including protein, calcium, and essential fats. The other two nutrients are Vitamin D, which our bodies make when we are exposed to the sun, and B_{12}, which is made from bacteria.[3] When we stop consuming poisonous substances like meat and dairy and swap them for nutrient dense starches such as health promoting fruits and veggies, the body will have the best chance to heal itself.[1,4]

McFact: Your body may even heal from so-called incurable diseases.
Given the right food, the body may even heal itself from diseases that doctors have categorized as "incurable".[1,4]

McFact: You don't have to count calories.
Dr. McDougall's dietary program, *The Starch Solution*, offers an easy approach to losing weight and regaining health.[5] Instead of restricting calories, the focus is on eating lots of whole nutritious foods, and skipping the junk food and animal products. You can eat all the food you want, but it has to be the right kind of food.

McFact: Get off your meds.
Most people in the first 10 days of following Dr. McDougall's program experience a drop in blood pressure and cholesterol. Most people are able to get off their drugs and medicines. The digestive system begins working optimally because it has the right food for the first time in years. If you keep going indefinitely with this lifestyle, your long term prognosis is a steady improvement in health and weight.[1,5]

McFact: You will gain a sense of well-being.
People who are eating a whole food, plant-based diet are found to have better moods and report higher levels of happiness.[6-8]

McFact: Eat when you are hungry.
You are not going to feel deprived on *The Starch Solution* program because you can eat when you are hungry and do not have to limit the quantity of the foods you eat. You just have to eat the right kinds of foods, and, get a load of this - it's the kind of food you love to eat naturally that your body is actually craving. It is food like mashed

potatoes and gravy, rice, pasta, and whole grain bread.[9]

McFact: Most diets fail.
The reason a lot of diets fail is because most of them are about restricting calories. Feeling hungry and feeling deprived is a lousy way to live your life and is something most people cannot sustain for long periods of time. The kicker is you usually regain all the weight back when you stop the diet and then some.[10,11]

McFact: Food can be a powerful medicine.
Food is the most powerful medicine on earth and you are getting three doses of it daily at breakfast, lunch, and dinner. Food can make you well or it can make you sick. In most cases, food is the only thing that can actually cure your serious ailments.[1,4]

McFact: Many vegans aren't healthy.
A lot of vegans are fat. This is because most vegans get the bulk of their calories from fat and protein just like they did when they ate the standard Western diet. If they switched to a starch-centered, oil-free diet, they would get their health and appearance back by dropping the extra pounds naturally.[12] People embracing the vegan lifestyle have already accomplished the most difficult hurdle, and that is eliminating meat and dairy from their diet. Now, it is important to embrace a healthy way to eat.

McFact: To stay healthy and well, follow this lifestyle for the rest of your life.
Once you understand how easy *The Starch Solution* program is, you can stay on it for long periods of time.[5] In fact, you could easily follow it for the rest of your life, and a lot of people do. Once you learn how to follow the program, it takes little effort to carry on with this healthy lifestyle. As chronic diseases disappear, as all that weight falls off, and you're having limitless amounts of energy, you won't want to go back to your old lifestyle ever again.

McFact: You have to decide if you are worth the effort.
Committing to a starch-centered diet, a daily walk, and developing healthy habits requires some focus, planning and effort, especially in the first several weeks. You are worth making the effort for improved health and longevity. If your life is at risk, it's time to make the change and turn things around.[1,4,5]

McFact: Your hunger drive is an almighty survival mechanism.
You can't fool it. It's a monster. Willpower cannot override your hunger drive. Your hunger drive will tell you that salad you had for dinner didn't cut it. Or, if you had half a sandwich, it will still leave you hungry. Whatever you try, you will never be comfortable with the discomfort of hunger.[13-15]

Reversing Disease

McFact: You can reverse many diseases with a starch-centered diet.
In addition to overcoming obesity, you can reverse serious, chronic, life-threatening illnesses like heart disease, high blood pressure, high cholesterol, diabetes, and arthritis. When you follow *The Starch Solution* program, many chronic conditions simply resolve and disappear. A whole food, starch-centered diet improves blood flow to all your organs and tissues. This means your skin is going to improve, and will no longer look or feel greasy. As your circulation improves, bringing nutrients and oxygen to every cell of your body, acne and other skin problems clear up, and aches and pains disappear.[16, 17]

McFact: There are many reports of spontaneous recovery from eating starch.
People who eat only healthy plant foods have reported spontaneous recovery from cancerous tumours affecting brain, colon, breast, skin, prostate, and kidney. People who eat only plant-based food have reported spontaneous recovery from other conditions as well, such as diabetes, hypertension, gallbladder pain, asthma, inflammation, high cholesterol, chronic diarrhea, constipation, and obesity.[1, 2, 4]

McFact: Starches do not contain dangerous toxic substances.
Unlike meat, starches don't contain toxic substances like cholesterol, saturated or trans fats, animal protein, dietary acid, chemical poisons, hormones, or pathogens that cause diseases. These are all present in meat and dairy and they are probably making you sick.[18-21]

The Miracles of Starch

McFact: Eat lots of potatoes, yams, corn rice and beans.

The main foods you should be eating are starches. Starches are your body's natural fuel. Starch breaks down into simple sugars. These sugars are what naturally feeds our body's systems and fuels our brain. Eating starches satisfies the appetite and keeps you feeling full for a long period of time.[5] As Dr. McDougall so clearly states about *The Starch Solution*, "You will look better, feel better, function better and live better! You will shed those pounds almost effortlessly!"[5]

Starchy plant foods fuel our bodies and provide us with complete proteins, omega-3 and 6 fatty acids, and the perfect blend of nutrients. With starch as the main fuel, our bodies will operate at optimal levels. The extra bonus is starch foods do not convert to fat.[22]

McFact: You can live on potatoes.
Potatoes and sweet potatoes are complete foods nutritionally. You can live on them for long periods of time. Historically, in times of famine and war that is exactly what our ancestors did. If you had only potatoes to eat, you would still be healthy and feel great.[23,24]

McFact: Carbs and starches do not make you fat.
Potatoes, rice, and whole grains do not turn to fat. As long as you are oil free, you will not get fat from eating starch! Even if you try to eat too many starches, your body will transform them into heat and energy rather than convert them into fat.[22] If you want to get healthy fast, eat potatoes, rice, and whole grains. Starches provide complete nutrition that enables the body to naturally heal itself and create continuous health. Starches have been vilified, and it is time for the truth to be known. They are full of plant protein, fibre, essential fatty acids, vitamins and minerals, phytates, and other phytochemicals and trace nutrients.[23,24]

The sugars in starch do not easily change to fat in humans. The complex carbohydrates of starchy foods are turned into simple sugars. These sugars are then transferred to the bloodstream and transported all over the body for fuel to trillions of cells. Your body can store up to two pounds of excess sugar in the muscles and liver. This sugar is called glycogen. The body will use this extra energy later as you move, or burn it as heat.[22]

McFACT: Even white flour and processed starches only turn into a small amount of fat.

Large quantities of white flour, refined and processed starches only convert to a small amount of body fat. They are stored in the body's muscles and later burned as energy.[22] It is the oil, margarines, and butter that you have to watch out for in refined baked goods and junk food that makes you fat.[25]

McFact: Starches are satisfying!
The taste buds on the tip of your tongue are excited by the starches you eat. They release hormones that cause neurological changes in your body, creating the sensation of contentment. We know bread, potatoes, and pasta are the comfort foods we love because of the way they make us feel.[13]

McFact: Fill your stomach with starches.
This is one of the ways to satisfy your hunger drive. Starches yield roughly one calorie per gram, while cheese and meat generate four calories per gram. Oil generates nine calories per gram. Starch not only makes you feel satisfied, it fills your stomach with a quarter of the number of calories.[13] You stay satisfied for a long time.

McFact: Starches provide the perfect amount of fat.
Fruits, starches, and vegetables have a small amount of natural fat. These plant foods are made of about 8 percent fat, enough to give you your perfect daily requirements of healthy fats. You do not need to add more fat to create a healthy diet.[13]

McFact: Carbohydrates and starches make your body happy.
Starchy foods are plants that are high in long chain digestible complex carbohydrates. You can eat unlimited quantities of whole grains like barley, wheat, corn, and rice. You can eat vegetables that are high in starch like squash, potatoes, sweet potatoes, and legumes like lentils, green peas, and beans.[13]

McFact: Humans are starchivores.
The scientific evidence is now showing that human beings are primarily starch eaters, and that they always have been. "Starchivore" would be an appropriate name for human beings. Carnivore for your cat. Herbivore for your horse. Starchivore for you.[26]

McFact: You need starch to feel good.
Although fruits, as well as green and yellow vegetables are important

and are packed full of nutrients, they do not provide enough calories to meet your daily energy demands. You must have enough calories to operate your brain, anatomy and physiology. You must eat starch to meet your daily energy demands.[13]

McFact: We have many starch taste buds on our tongue.
In our saliva, amylase is the enzyme that breaks down starch into simple sugars. It has been found that human saliva has six to eight times more of this starch digesting enzyme, amylase, than the lesser primates. This data shows that among primates, humans are designed to eat a starch-based diet.[27]

Meat, Eggs, and Dairy Make You Fat and Sick

McFact: The rich were always fat and sick.
With the onset of the Industrial Revolution, never in the history of the world have large populations of people had the income to buy meat, eggs, and milk as a dietary staple. Before this, it was only the rich who could afford these luxuries, and it was only the rich who had degenerative diseases and obesity. These are now the same diseases that plague modern humans.[28]

McFact: Meat is a food poison.
Beef, poultry, fish, seafood, dairy and eggs are food poison and are the leading cause illness in human beings. They will often make you sick and can cause you to die prematurely.[19]

For those who are determined to keep eating meat and dairy, they are at increased risk of developing chronic illnesses, obesity, and premature death. Every time you eat these things, you injure your body. In fact, you are injuring your body three times a day, with breakfast, lunch and dinner! As soon as you stop eating these foods, your body has the ability to start to heal itself because you have stopped the harmful behavior.[19]

McFact: You can reduce your risk of disease by 90 percent.
Scientists have found that if you eat a diet of whole plant foods and starches, and by skipping the meat and dairy products, the chances of you getting degenerative illnesses are reduced by 90 percent.[1,4,5]

McFact: Most people don't know that meat and dairy are dangerous.
Most people don't realize and are unaware that meat and dairy products are poisonous and are likely to make you sick. People are misguided by advertising and big businesses, having us believe that they are an essential part of a healthy diet.

McFact: We don't need high amounts of protein to be healthy.
The World Health Organization recommends that only five percent of our daily calories need to come from protein. For an average man, this would be 38 grams per day for a diet of 3000 calories. For women it would be 29 grams per day for an average diet of 2300 calories.[29] We can easily get the perfect amount of our daily protein needs from eating whole food starches and vegetables.

McFact: Eating too much animal protein is dangerous.
Excess animal protein can induce low energy, cause osteoporosis, kidney damage and kidney stones, promote tumour growth, cause arthritis and other inflammatory diseases.[19] Meat when digested is acidic. Eating too much meat compromises the immune function and makes the body prone to the attack of viruses and bacteria.[19,30,31]

McFact: It doesn't matter if the meat is free range and organic, it can still cause disease.
All animal foods can cause illness whether the food was raised in a large factory farm using antibiotics and chemicals or grown organically and/or free range in your backyard.[32]

McFact: All meat and dairy products are equally bad for you.
It doesn't matter if it is the flesh of a cow, chicken, duck, goat, lamb or fish. White meat is not healthier. Fish is not healthier. It doesn't matter if it is the milk and cheese from a cow, or a goat. All animal foods are comprised of a combination of high levels of animal protein, animal fat, and cholesterol. These foods contain large amounts of sulfur-carrying amino acid methionine as well as harmful dietary acids.[32]

McFact: Cholesterol is almost entirely found in animal foods.
Overtime, it becomes difficult for our bodies to get rid of the excess cholesterol from animal foods and that becomes a real problem. High blood cholesterol is a marker for heart disease and dementia among other things. Cholesterol also aids in the development of cancer.[32]

A serving size of 3.5 ounces of the following foods yields the following cholesterol levels:

Type of Food	Beef	Pork	Shrimp	Skinned Chicken Breast	Tofu	Pinto Beans
Cholesterol Levels	89 mg	90 mg	194 mg	85 mg	0 mg	0 mg

Source: ucsfhealth.org/education/cholesterol_content_of_foods/

McFact: Homocysteine levels increase when you eat meat.
Increased homocysteine levels show that you are at higher risk for a heart attack, stroke, thrombosis, dementia, Alzheimer's or depression.[33]

McFact: Animal foods are linked to increased tumor growth.
Dr. T. Colin Campbell has shown that consuming more than eight percent animal protein turns cancer growth on. To reduce your risk of cancer, limit animal protein in your daily diet to below eight percent. Or better yet, don't eat animal foods at all.[34]

McFact: Meat is full of fattening saturated fat.
Animal fat is one of the most dangerous kinds of fat because it is saturated fat, causing heart disease, stroke, and artery damage. Beef is 60 to 80 percent saturated fat; pork is 80 to 95 percent saturated fat; chicken is 30 to 50 percent saturated fat; and fish is up to 60 percent saturated fat. Animal fat is toxic.[32]

In North America, 68 percent of adults are now overweight. Our bodies store fat easily. The animal fat you eat at every meal goes directly to your buttocks, hips, thighs, and stomach, and is making you fatter after every meal.[32]

Excess fat is also deposited in and around our organs like our liver, heart, and muscles. The collection of fat in these organs is a marker for a state called insulin resistance. This fatty state is an indicator that heart disease, stroke, and type 2 diabetes are on your doorstep.[35]

McFact: Science shows that you don't need to eat meat for optimal health.
Many scientific studies now show animal products are not a necessary part of a healthy diet, and can increase your risk of disease.[36]

McFact: Processed meat is a carcinogen.
After compiling the results of more than 800 studies, the World Health Organization (WHO) announced on October 26th, 2015, that processed meats, such as ham and sausages, can cause colon, stomach, and other cancers. WHO also stated that red meat most likely causes cancer, and categorized processed meats in the same danger category as cigarettes and asbestos.[37]

Protein and Calcium

McFact: Plant foods are packed with protein.
Plant proteins found in rice and potatoes provide all the protein and essential amino acids you and your children need.[4, 23, 24] Based on the latest scientific data, people are eating too much protein. A person only has a protein requirement of about 20-30 grams daily. Plant foods can easily provide that amount. In a typical Western diet, most people over eat proteins, getting 100 to 160 grams per day. Dr. McDougall recommends 30-60 grams per day.[32]

McFact: Protein from animals is not superior to protein from plants.
Some of the most powerful and muscular animals on earth are plant eaters. Your average muscular elephant, hippopotamus, giraffe, and horse eat only plants, and they all achieve their daily protein requirements. It only seems logical that you can too.[36]

McFact: Animal proteins are different from plant proteins.
Animal proteins contain amino acids that have a sulfa compound which is toxic to our liver and kidneys. When you are suffering from kidney or liver disease, your doctor usually puts you on a low animal protein diet. This gives your kidneys and liver a chance to heal.[38]

McFact: Get your calcium from plants.
Calcium doesn't originate in cow's milk. Where does the cow get the calcium that is in her milk? The plants the cow eats absorb calcium and other minerals through their roots. You can skip drinking the cow's milk and go right to the plant source to get your calcium.[39]

Plants have just as much usable calcium as cow's milk. Eat some broccoli instead. One cup of milk has 300 mg of calcium, and one cup of cooked collard greens has 360 mg of calcium! One cup of cooked kale has 210 mg of calcium.[39]

McFact: There are no diseases in modern man related to calcium deficiency.
The dairy industry has duped you into believing you will have a calcium shortage and get sick if you don't drink their milk.[39]

McFact: That glass of milk may actually be harming your bones.
Scientific evidence is showing that people who drink the most milk and eat the most cheese and yogurt have the highest rates of osteoporosis and hip fractures later in life.[40]

McFact: Skim milk is fattening.
Even though the milk is labelled low-fat or skim, it still contains one third (32 percent) of its calories from fat.[40]

McFact: Cheese is almost pure fat.
Cheese has a total of 70 percent of calories coming from saturated and trans fats.[40] Cheese is made from the fat that has been removed from the milk to make it "skim".

McFact: Dairy is a main source of estrogen and linked to cancers of the breast, uterus, and prostate.
About 60 to 70 percent of estrogens found in the Standard American Diet come from dairy foods. As a consequence, cancers of the breast, uterus and prostate have been positively associated with the consumption of dairy.[40]

Lose All of Your Excess Weight

McFact: Eating fat is one of the main causes of obesity and type 2 diabetes.
Globally, in first world countries, 68 percent of people are overweight. Worldwide, 371 million people suffer from type 2 diabetes. The average American eats 23 pounds of cheese yearly, and the average European eats 17.2 kilograms of cheese yearly. These amounts are three times what people ate in 1970![41]

McFact: Lose Weight by Eating Starch.
The fat falls off your body easily when you eat the McDougall way.

Eating a diet high in starches causes you to lose excess body fat. You get your looks back as you reach and maintain your optimal weight. You will have loads of energy, and a positive sense of well-being.[4, 5, 13]

McFact: In the United States, 38 percent of adults are obese.
While 68 percent of people in North America are overweight, 80 percent of adults in the United States are carrying excess weight, and 38 percent of Americans are obese. Being overweight and obese from eating rich junk foods leads to all sorts of terrible health issues. You feel lethargic and down on yourself for not having more willpower.[13] When you follow Dr. McDougall's starch-centered plan, you will discover this is not about willpower, this is about eating the right kind of food.

Eating Oils and Fats are Bad for Your Health

McFact: We get all the fat we need from plants.
The human body requires omega-3 and omega-6 essential fats. They are called essential because we cannot produce them ourselves and must get them from the foods we eat. We can get all the fats we need from whole plant foods without adding extra oil. All plants make these essential fats and they comprise about eight percent of each plant. They also make 11 of the 13 essential nutrients we require. Sun exposure and bacteria make the missing two, which are vitamins D and B_{12}. These fats make cell membranes and synthesize hormones. Humans, animals, and fish can't make their own omega-3 and omega-6 fatty acids. Like us, they must get them from the food they eat.[42]

McFact: Don't put any more oil in your food.
It is important not to eat any extra fat in your diet. When we eat fat daily, the body can easily take the fat from the food and within hours of consumption, store it in our cells.[42]

McFact: The fat in high fat foods makes you fat.
When you eat any high fat foods like dairy, meat, eggs, fish, nuts and seeds, animal and vegetable oils, the body transfers the fat from your intestines into your bloodstream where it is transported to the billions of fat storage cells called adipose cells. Your body does this transfer effortlessly after every fat-filled meal.[42]

McFact: Olive oil, margarine, and all vegetable oils are not healthy.
Olive oil and non-dairy margarine made from plants are just as high in fat as animal products and they cause just as much damage. They easily become the fat stored on your thighs, hips, and stomach. Vegetable oils are just as dangerous as animal fats at advancing cancer. Blood clots that form inside the arteries are what cause most heart attacks. The science reveals that in long term studies, olive oil increases blood clotting just as much as animal fat does.[42]

McFact: You get tired after you eat fats and oils.
Fats and oils reduce blood oxygen and impair circulation by a factor of 20 percent. This can cause chest pain, diminished brain function, high blood pressure, weariness, and weakened lung function.[42]

McFact: Nuts and seeds are fattening.
Nuts and seeds are full of protein, vitamins and thousands of trace nutrients. About 80 percent of their calories come from fat, which is why you are recommended to limit yourself to one ounce of nuts and seeds per day to avoid oily skin and weight gain.[42] For those who wish to lose weight, it is best to avoid nuts and seeds altogether.

Dairy is Not Meant for Human Consumption

McFact: Dairy increases IGF-1 levels in humans.
The primary protein in milk and cheese is called casein, and when consumed, can increase the liver's production of the growth hormone IGF-1, which has been shown to increase tumour growth in breast, prostate, colon, brain, and lung cancers.[43]

McFact: Milk and dairy products make us fat and sick.
Nature never intended human children or adults to drink cow's milk. It is full of compounds that can make you fat and sick. Dairy products often cause food allergies and some autoimmune diseases like asthma, arthritis, and multiple sclerosis (MS). Cow's milk is for calves.[43]

McFact: Dairy is dangerous.
Out of all the foods, dairy products are recalled most often because they are repeatedly tainted with pathogens. These pathogens, bacteria and microbes like salmonella, staphylococci, listeria, and e-coli, can

cause life-threatening infections. They may also contain viruses that cause lymphoma and leukemia-like diseases.[44]

Fish is Not Healthy for You

McFact: Most people believe that fish is healthy.
They believe fish is a source of good fats. Actually, the fish get these essential fats from eating seaweed and algae. You can get them too by bypassing the fish and eating the plants instead.[45]

McFact: Eating fish is hazardous to your health.
Fish is polluted with toxic chemicals like methyl-mercury, PCBs and DDT. Salmon, tuna, mackerel, sardines, pike, walleye, and bass are all at the top of the food chain and are highly toxic, and may cause brain damage and cancer.[45] Taking fish oil supplements and eating oily fish does not reduce the incidence of heart attack and other cardiovascular events, nor do they reduce the incidence of cancer.[46]

McFact: Seafood may cause mercury poisoning in humans.
Seafood is contaminated with toxic levels of mercury and is the number one cause of chronic mercury poisoning in humans. You can damage your heart, kidneys, immune and nervous systems from mercury poisoning. Mercury poisoning can also affect the brain causing all sorts of havoc like interruptions in motor function, loss of memory, learning disabilities, and depression.[45]

McFact: Eating fish may increase your risk of cardiovascular disease.
The mercury poisoning present in fish affects the brain and kidneys, and also damages the blood vessels. Inflammation, blood clots, interruptions in muscle function can all occur in the blood vessel walls from mercury poisoning and lead to cardiovascular disease. Skip the fish and get omega-3 fats from plant foods.[45]

Growth Hormone IGF-1 and Tumour Growth

McFact: Isolated soy protein products are dangerous.
These foods are processed and the protein is extracted from the whole bean. Soy foods such as fake meat products are refined and lack all the key components that make that food healthy: like fibre, carbohydrates,

fat, vitamins, minerals and trace nutrients. Once the food is refined, it can cause an increased growth in cancerous tumours because it increases the liver's production of IGF-1.[47]

McFact: Eating Meat and Dairy accelerates aging.
Milk, as well as meat, shell fish, eggs, and soy protein isolates, all increase the production of growth hormones and specifically IGF-1, which accelerates aging. Telomeres, the caps at the end of each strand of DNA that protect our chromosomes, will shorten as we age. There is now research showing that by following a healthy plant-based diet, telomeres will lengthen.[48] This indicates that we can extend our lives by changing what we eat. If you want to live a longer, healthier life, get rid of the red meat, pork, poultry, fish, eggs and dairy.[40, 46]

Vitamin Supplements

McFact: Take a B_{12} supplement on a starch-centered diet.
People who are eating a plant-based diet need to take five micrograms of B_{12} daily.[49] B_{12} is made from a microbe that is found on plant foods. Since this is not the safest way to get our B_{12} needs met, it is best to take a supplement.

McFact: You will get enough nutrients from plant food.
When you eat a whole food plant-based diet, you are getting all of your essential proteins, vitamins, minerals and trace nutrients. Unless you have a health issue that is not affected by the change to a healthy, starch-centered diet, you do not need to take vitamin supplements. There is no shortage of nutrients in a plant-based diet.[50]

McFact: People worry there is a mineral deficiency in our depleted soils.
The chances of this happening are extremely small. Our day-to-day fruits and vegetables are imported from different farms from all over the world. This week your oranges could be from Spain, Mexico, or Chile, and grown in a wide variety of soils. It is just a sales pitch to get you to buy vitamins from the vitamin industry.[51]

McFact: People take supplements out of fear.
People fear that they are not getting enough nutrients from their diet, and hope they can prevent or cure an illness by popping vitamin pills.

The most complete natural nutrients are in whole plant-based foods, not supplements.[51]

The Truth About Sugar

McFact: Sugar does not make you fat or sick.
Eating fat is the real cause of weight gain and sickness, not sugar. There is unjustifiable fear of sugar being the cause of the worldwide epidemic of type 2 diabetes, cancer, obesity, arthritis, heart disease, and intestinal disorders. This is simply not true as the science shows. Instead of being afraid of sugar, you should really be wary of fat, oil, and animal products in your diet. That is where the true problem lies.[52]

McFact: You can eat a little sugar.
The giant modification that you have made to stop eating animal foods, junk food and foods laced with fats to a starch-centred diet is a giant step towards getting your health back. If a teaspoon of brown sugar will help you switch to eating oatmeal for breakfast, then Dr. McDougall wants you to look forward to your first meal of the day. A teaspoon of brown sugar is just 16 calories, which will not cause you to gain any weight. It could, however, make you enjoy eating your food much more*.[52]

*However, if sugar is a food that triggers your cravings for more sugary and sweet foods, then it is best to avoid it. You could try replacing the sugar on your oatmeal with cinnamon. Cinnamon has a surprisingly sweet flavor.

McFact: Sugar does not cause type 2 diabetes.
The scientific community now recognizes that type 2 diabetes is not caused by eating sugar and carbohydrates. Sugar has been misjudged as the primary cause of many diseases, including obesity, and has often been used as the scapegoat to conceal the true culprits, the meat and dairy industries. This does not mean, however, that white processed sugar and flour, the main ingredients in junk food products, are healthy choices. Overeating sugar and flour laden junk foods will lead to obesity and poor health*.[52]

*If sugar consumption in any amount triggers addictive tendencies for you, please avoid it altogether. This includes agave nectar, maple syrup, rice syrup, coconut sugar, stevia, dried fruits (raisins and the like), honey, dates, figs, and any artificial sweeteners like xylitol, aspartame, and saccharin.

McFact: Refined sugars and flours cause undernourishment.

For a lot of people in our modern world, they may eat mostly candy bars, cookies, crackers, and white bread. These foods have been stripped of all their nutrient value in manufacturing. These "empty calorie" foods are consumed in vast quantities, rendering the average person malnourished.[53]

Most Doctors Don't Acknowledge the Importance of Nutritional Science

McFact: Many medical doctors know very little about nutrition.

It is not on the curriculum of a number of medical schools, and if it is, it is estimated to be an average of 19 hours of nutritional education in the entire four years of medical training. It is an anomaly in our society that your own doctor has little to no idea what you should be eating to prevent, treat, or remedy the leading causes of illness.[54,55] Doctors are just as easily influenced by the media and propaganda from the drug and food organizations posing as authorities as the general public. It is a shame that they do not have this powerful tool for preventing and treating disease in their medical tool kits.

The Political Dilemma

McFact: Your government is not necessarily looking out for your health.

The governments and ruling agencies should be watching out for the best interest of the public. Unfortunately, the system is flawed. Governments have allegiances and loyalties to big agribusinesses, leaving you to figure out what is good for you on your own.[56]

McFact: Advertising does not tell the truth.

The big agricultural businesses have millions of dollars to spend enrolling us and our children with slick advertising campaigns. People mistake what they hear in these advertisements as the truth. With so much misinformation floating around, how can a consumer really know what products are healthy for him and his family? What you hear and read in the media about health food is not necessarily the truth. Go to drmcdougall.com or nutritionfacts.org for the truth about food and nutrition.

McFact: Your food choices are influenced by the bottom line.
The multi-million-dollar TV ads say it's healthy. The government, which is supposed to be protecting us, has loyalties to the big agribusinesses first, says it is healthy. That doesn't make it so. As an example, there are a lot of big businesses who don't want you and your family to stop drinking milk because there are big profits to be made. At what expense? You and your family's health and well-being. As a result, never before in the history of humankind has there been such a critical epidemic of fat and sick people.[28, 57]

McFact: What is good for industry is not necessarily good for you.
They don't seem to care if you get sick from their products, rather they only seem to care about their bottom line. Dr. McDougall said in a recent interview, "We need the people in this country to know the truth and know the food industry is killing us, and the heart surgery industry and oncology industry are killing us. We will look back someday and realize that this is the most ugly, vicious thing that human beings have ever done to each other, ever."[58]

Our World is Worth Saving

McFact: You are making a difference when you eat a starch-centered diet.
When you decide to improve your health by eating a whole food plant-based diet you will automatically become an environmentalist and contribute to healing the planet with absolutely no added effort.[59] You see, you are no longer contributing to the production of meat, which is the leading cause of world greenhouse gases.

McFact: Raising animals causes global warming.
The production of animal foods in factory farms is one of the leading causes of climate change and global warming. The enormous quantities of animals that are being raised and slaughtered are causing the most damage to our environment.[59] It is hard to imagine the expansive scale of meat production in the world, but it has become a threat to our

environment. In the United States alone, 11 billion animals are slaughtered each year to feed meat eaters.[60]

McFact: It takes a lot of resources to raise meat.
To raise one pound of beef takes 12 pounds of grain, 55 square feet of rainforest, and 2500 gallons of water. To make one pound of pork takes four pounds of grain, and takes two pounds of grain to make one pound of chicken. If everybody stopped eating meat, we would have enough food to feed everybody in the world.[61]

McFact: Eating a diet free of animal foods will be the single biggest thing you can do to help the environment.
Factory farming, the raising of animals for people to eat, causes fifty-one percent of global greenhouse gases. The animal foods industry is the largest contributor to climate change and many are saying it is killing our planet. The irony is a diet that is high in animal protein is probably killing you too.[59]

McFact: The fish are disappearing.
Since 1950, the number of fish in our lakes, rivers, and oceans have been reduced by ninety percent by the fishing industry. All sea life is struggling, with populations diminishing at an alarming rate. The Bluefin tuna, Atlantic cod, Alaskan king crab, and Pacific salmon are almost extinct. There are many other species that no longer exist. This is a grave situation. Only 10 percent of the fish population is left on planet Earth compared to what was available in 1950. The last of the fish are being wiped out by people who are misinformed, believing that eating fish is healthy.[45]

McFact: Our world is worth saving.
Planet Earth is the only home we have, and we must act now to save ourselves from extinction. You are worth it. Your children and grandchildren are worth it.

Chapter Four

No Longer Fat, Sick and Hungry
Dr. John McDougall's Program

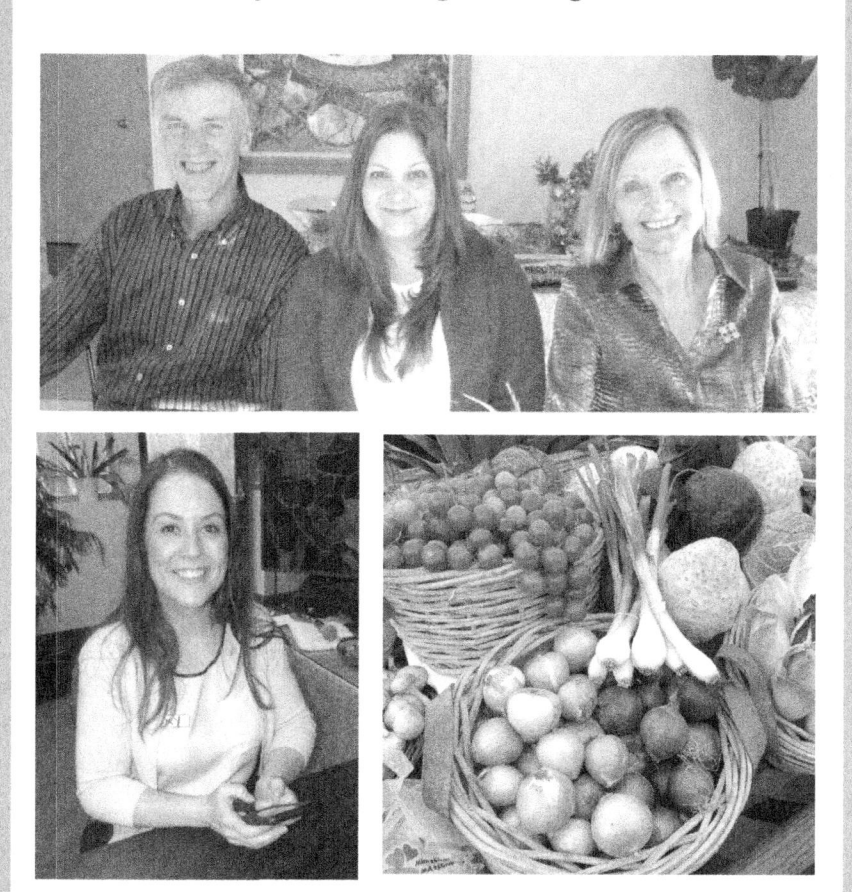

Toronto Starch Solution Meetup Group

Chapter Four - Dr. John McDougall's Program

No Longer Fat, Sick, and Hungry

Are you ready to lose some weight and get healthy? If so, then your life is about to improve in so many wonderful ways. From now on, the only foods you are going to be eating are plant-based foods. This means that all foods from the animal kingdom will no longer be in your diet. The bulk of your calories, 70 to 90 percent of them, will be coming from complex carbohydrates, also known as starchy vegetables like potatoes, whole intact grains such as brown rice and quinoa, and beans. Your body requires starches to generate enough energy and nutrition to optimally operate all your physiological systems. These starchy foods will give you vitality, energy, and strength. Your mental health and level of happiness will improve as well.[1-4]

As well as potatoes, grains, and beans, you may eat whole grain products such as multigrain or sprouted breads, whole grain pastas, corn tortillas, and whole grain cereals like steel cut oats. Also in the starch category are many kinds of root vegetables like potatoes and sweet potatoes. Unless there is a risk that sugar or salt will trigger overeating in yourself, Dr. McDougall allows you to add a sprinkle of salt or sugar to the surface of your food without compromising your health. You will find the starches to be delicious, filling and satisfying.

Fed Up with Being Fat and Sick

The best part of this program is that you never feel deprived. If you get hungry you can eat as much starch as you want. In fact, you'll never get tired of eating starchy foods because they're the best fuel for your body. Additionally, you can eat a variety of fruits and vegetables, and add an assortment of herbs and spices to the many delicious vegetable dishes that you can enjoy to your heart's content.

To recap, the only foods you will be eating are going to be plant-based foods. Exclude all animal products including dairy products (milk, cream, cheese, yogurt, sour cream, ricotta, cream cheese, ice cream and butter), eggs, fish, shellfish, and all the meats and flesh of animals of every kind. You'll follow the plant-based rule of never eating anything that has a face or a mother.

The last food category you need to eliminate to obtain optimal health, are all of the oils. Trust us, when we say you eliminate oils, this means all of them! All oils are equally damaging and this includes olive oil, safflower oil and corn oil.[9-13] Olive oil is not healthy! To avoid the ill effects from consuming oil, you will now use water or vegetable broth instead of oil or butter when sautéing or "frying". (We like to call it "water frying".) Salad dressings and baked goods must also be oil-free.

For those of you who struggle, who fight the cravings for pizza, burgers, fries, ice cream and cake, please read *The Pleasure Trap* by Drs. Lisle and Goldhamer.[14] Read it at least twice. Remove the temptations you have in your fridge and kitchen cupboards. Ask those you live with to hide their food, in a locked cupboard if necessary. Ask them to go out to eat at restaurants if they wish to have the food you cannot eat. Do everything you can to keep your home free of the food that will tempt you.

Dr. McDougall recommends that you contact your doctor and let him or her know that you are treating your ailments with a whole food, plant-based, starch-centered diet. Your doctor will have to monitor your medications and in many cases, reduce or even eliminate them as you grow healthier and thinner. Keep in mind that your doctor may find it difficult to believe that you can actually heal yourself by eating a nutritious diet of plant foods. In a 2015 survey of US medical schools, the average amount of time spent on nutrition education is 19 hours in the entire four years of an MD program.[15]

This starch-centered approach is also not information the average person may be willing to accept as true. Don't let the scepticism of your friends, family and coworkers, influence, discourage, or negatively affect you. You are learning about the power of plant foods to heal the human body. You are learning about the ability of a starch-centered diet to put serious health issues into remission, backed by scientific research. You can set the example to your doctor, family and friends, and be the change you want to be.

When you are starting this plan, get a blood workup from your doctor. You might find it helpful to keep a record of your progress. Write down your starting weight and lab results. Keep track of what you eat and how much you exercise. Record your initial symptoms and note when they start to disappear. Take note of your mood and energy levels when you begin and document any improvements as you go along.

When you first begin, even if your blood work is in the normal range, it doesn't mean that you are healthy. You may be at the low end or high end of what is considered normal, but it is usually just a matter of time before your blood work shows you are unhealthy. For example, your blood glucose may be in the normal range, but if it's at the high end of normal, you may be in the first stages of insulin resistance. Without dietary and lifestyle changes you may soon be dealing with type 2 diabetes.

From Dr. McDougall's website, drmcdougall.com:

Take your blood pressure and get your blood test results, including the five following measurements:

1. Have your doctor check your cholesterol. If it is too high, it is a warning sign for circulatory problems that can lead to heart attack, stroke, or dementia. This program will naturally improve your cholesterol without medications. If you are taking medicine for high cholesterol, you doctor is going to have to monitor, reduce, and very likely have you stop taking your medication.

2. Check your triglycerides, which point out the density of the fat particles that are circulating in your blood. Higher amounts of fat in your blood shows you are at risk for type 2 diabetes and

heart disease.

3. Have your glucose (blood sugar) levels checked. This is another indicator for pre-diabetes or diabetes.

4. Have your BUN (blood urea nitrogen) checked. This test reveals the amount of protein you eat and the impact that it is having on your kidneys. Your doctor will tell you if it is within a normal range.

5. Have your uric acid level checked. If these levels are too high, you are at risk of having gout or kidney stones.

Document all of your medications, and under your doctor's supervision, track the reduction in amounts of medication you take and also the drugs you eliminate as you progress. You can also take body measurements when you begin, and take them again as you move to your optimal weight and health.

Dr. McDougall points out that the hardest part of this program, by far, is just getting started.[4] For many people, they need a compelling reason to try it. It could be a life-threatening situation like heart disease, cancer, or chronic pain that drives you to follow this way of eating. Perhaps, you have a parent that went through a painful death and you don't want to experience the same thing. Maybe you're just sick and tired of being overweight. Whatever your reasons are, just remember, the hardest part is just starting. Once you begin feeling better, you won't want to stop. Your body wants to be healthy and when you give it the optimal nutrition it needs, it can begin to repair the damage and heal on its own.

Get Ready...Get Set....GO!

Before you begin, make some preparations and do some research. Set some goals. What would you like to accomplish in the first 10 days? Perhaps it will be the reduction of chest pain, and the ability to breathe easier. Perhaps, it will be to lose weight, or cut down on your insulin. Maybe you are hoping for your arthritic pain to ease up or to get off some of your medications. Make a commitment to do this program and be all in so you can enjoy the rewards and see for yourself that it really works.

The next step is to research what you would like to eat. A good place to find recipes is on Dr. McDougall's website, drmcdougall.com. Mary McDougall has created over 2000 oil-free recipes, and we can tell you they're all delicious. On the website, there is also a meal plan for a 10-day period. If you are stuck on what to eat for breakfast, lunch, and dinner, Mary and Dr. McDougall have it all worked out for you. You can also find recipes created by Mary McDougall in all of the 11 books she has co-written with her husband.

Now that you have decided what you are going to eat, make your shopping list, and hit the grocery store. Stock your kitchen with your new foods. Plan on packing lunches to bring with you to work or when you are out for the day, and carry lots of snacks. You never know when your monster hunger drive will show up - you don't want to get caught without energy packed starches! By planning ahead and being prepared, your chances of success will be much higher.

Don't forget to clean out your fridge, freezer, and cupboards of all the taboo foods. Do this to make your home environment a McDougall-approved zone. This way, there won't be any foods that will tempt you in weak moments as you transition to this new way of eating. If you live with others, then it will be important to sit down with them and work out what you need to be successful. If you're one of the lucky ones, you may be able to turn your whole kitchen into a McDougall paradise! However, if your family or your housemates are not open to such a change, then you will need to set aside areas that allow for other foods that you must stay away from.

You are probably going to want to tell your family and friends about your decision to begin this program. Hopefully, they will be supportive. People react in different ways. You might be pleasantly surprised that family members are on board and willing to support you and share your excitement for the new food and results you are getting. They may even decide to join you and get healthy and slim!

On the other hand, you might have to be tolerant of their anger and disappointment as you get slim and well, and they are not on that same path to better health. Sometimes loved ones, whether or not they realize they are sabotaging your efforts, will bring home foods you can't have, or will continue to make foods with oil. From our experience, it is best to not argue or get upset with a loved one about this. Simply repeat to them that this is no longer your food (animal foods, butters, margarines, and oils), and that eating *The Starch Solution* way is healing you and allowing you to live a longer, healthier life. You may have to take over with cooking your own meals 100 percent, but be sure to make enough for everyone in your home to enjoy with you. If they still choose to drizzle oil on their vegetables, so be it. Say nothing, just continue your path to better health and lead by example.

If you like to eat in restaurants, make a commitment to stick to the plant-based options. You can always find delicious dishes with vegetables only. The trick is to get the chef to prepare your food without oil. Be prepared to ask ahead of ordering your meal about keeping oil out of your food. It's often a good idea to call in advance and speak with someone from the kitchen. If there is resistance, it will help to say you are under doctor's orders to eat plant-based and avoid all fats and oils.

Caffeine, cigarettes, and alcohol are a detriment to good health, therefore Dr. McDougall advises that this is a good time to get them under control.[15] However, if you are not an all-or-nothing type of person, it's probably a good idea to do one thing at a time. Take the first 30 days to practice eating *The Starch Solution* way. Then, once you are feeling confident about the change in your eating habits, take a serious look at your caffeine intake and reduce it by half. Eventually, resolve to get it out of your daily life. If you're a smoker, work on cutting down and with time, quitting those cancer sticks. The same with alcohol, cut it down to a maximum of three drinks per week, and eventually cut it out. Your liver will love you and you will feel so much better.

Keeping It Simple

Food is a powerful medicine, and you are getting a powerful dose of that medicine three times a day at breakfast, lunch, and dinner! Healthy, whole plant food prevents the majority of diseases and will often heal existing ones. When you commit 100 percent to doing at least 30 days on *The Starch Solution* program, things are going to get better for your body. This is going to be the best gift you have ever given to yourself in your entire life!

Dr. McDougall's program is built on the foundation of eating starch. Of the food you eat, 70 to 90 percent will be made up of whole, unrefined starches, like oatmeal for breakfast, rice for lunch, and potatoes for dinner. To these starchy basics, you can add tasty fruits, vegetables, beans and legumes. By keeping it simple, you have a better chance of crossing over into a basic routine of preparing foods that you will enjoy throughout the day. Although there are a huge variety of fruits, vegetables and starches to choose from, Dr. McDougall's advice is to keep your choices very simple. Even if you choose the same things every day, you are assured you are getting the optimal amount of nutrients. Don't worry if you think you won't be getting enough protein. Plant foods are packed with protein.

One supplement you will need to eventually start taking is B_{12}. Depending on your current stores of Vitamin B_{12}, it could take as long as six years before you run out.[25] Rather than wait out those six years, it's probably better to take a B_{12} supplement weekly, and have your levels checked yearly by your doctor to see if you can remain with a weekly dose or if you should take it daily.

What You Can Eat on Dr. McDougall's Starch Solution Program

To begin with, eat lots of starchy vegetables, grains, beans and legumes that will fill you up and give you the energy requirements your body needs. Make these the center of each meal you eat. Here is a list of the foods you can enjoy:

- **Starchy root vegetables**. Eat lots of these. There are many delicious root vegetables such as sweet potatoes, white potatoes, and yams that contain the energy requirements to fuel our bodies. They all come in many interesting varieties and colours. Did you know you can live off white potatoes?[26] Potatoes have all the nutrients, trace elements, and starches to fuel and feed the human body without having to add anything else to your diet.

- **Winter squashes**. They are high in carbohydrates and are perfect for the center of your meal as they can provide enough fuel for your body: butternut, acorn, Hubbard, banana, pumpkin, buttercup, turban squash. The summer squashes, unlike winter squashes, tend to be low in calorie content so they are not considered a starch but are perfect to eat as a side dish.

- **Whole intact grains**. Eat plenty of these starches: corn, wheat, barley, rye, quinoa, oats, brown rice, wild rice, buckwheat, couscous, wheat berries, bulgur, and millet.

- **Pastas, breads, crackers, wraps**. The problem with these foods is that they are made from highly refined flours. If you are at a normal weight, then you can enjoy moderate portions. However, for those who need to lose weight, you are encouraged to avoid foods made from flours, including the breads and pastas made from whole wheat, brown rice, and other grains.

- **Root vegetables**. There are all kinds of root vegetables you can enjoy that are not considered a starch because they are low in carbohydrates and calories. These can make a delicious side dish: carrots, turnips, parsnips, beets, celery root, tapioca, Jerusalem artichoke, water chestnuts, daikon, and burdock.

- **Legumes, beans, and lentils**. Beans and lentils are the perfect starchy choice as the center of your meal. They include: garbanzo or chickpeas, black beans, lima beans, adzuki beans, mung beans, navy beans, fava beans, red kidney beans, pinto beans, cannellini beans, brown lentils, green lentils, red lentils, black-eyed peas, split green peas, whole green peas, split yellow peas. Even though soybeans have zero cholesterol, they are not included as a starch because they are 45 percent fat. If you are trying to lose weight, products like tofu and tempeh are best avoided due to their fat content.

- **Green and yellow vegetables**. Green and red pepper, celery, bok choy, radish, broccoli, tomatoes, spinach, lettuces, cucumber, zucchini, cauliflower, arugula, kale, burdock, radicchio, celeriac, chicory, Swiss chard, collard greens, taro root, water chestnuts, endive, watercress, sprouts (alfalfa, lentil, mung bean, wheat), Jerusalem artichoke, daikon. These vegetables are great for side dishes but are not starches and are low in calories. You can eat all the green and yellow vegetables you want with no limitations.

- **Fruits. There isn't a fruit that is off limits**: apples, oranges, peaches, pears, plums, berries, mango, bananas, kiwi fruit, grapes, papaya, pomegranate, passion fruit, kumquat, lychee and others. Although fruits are packed with all kinds of nutrients, they do contain a lot of simple sugars. Dr. McDougall suggests you limit yourself to three servings of fruit each day. Since they taste so good, it would be easy to over do it. Fructose is the main sugar in fruit and for some people, it causes triglycerides and cholesterol to go up.[16]

- **Nuts and seeds in small amounts**. These are nutrient dense foods but beware, they are packed with fat. Keep your portions to no more than a handful of nuts a day, and if you are trying to lose weight, avoid them altogether. Many low-fat milk alternatives are made from almond and cashew nuts, hemp seeds, and rice. They are great alternatives to put on your morning cereal or to use in your cooking. For example, they can be baked into casseroles.

In summary, there are many varieties of starches, fruits, and vegetables to try once you feel you are established on your starch-centered diet. Don't feel that it is mandatory to have a variety of fruits and vegetables on this program. Simple, repetitive food choices of starches with some vegetables and fruits will more than adequately sustain and meet all your nutritional needs.

Meat and Dairy are Hazardous to Your Health

Here is a list of animal products and a few plant foods that are not allowed on *The Starch Solution* program.

- **Meat**. Eliminate all meat from your diet including beef, pork, poultry, fish, seafood, wild game, along with soups and gravies made with animal stock. You should be no longer consuming any foods that have animal fat or proteins listed in the ingredients. These foods are very high in fat, contain dangerous additives, and have no fibre. They contain high amounts of cholesterol and are devoid of many essential vitamins and minerals. High levels of animal proteins promote disease.[17,18]

- Be aware that the vegan processed foods sold in stores is not whole plant-based food either. It is still processed food with chemical preservatives and cheap ingredients for the intention of making a quick profit. This would be things like processed meat substitutes, such as veggie dogs. Check the ingredients before you purchase any processed food. Remember, processed food is not whole plant food. Stick to whole foods, the ones you find in the produce section of your grocery store.

- **Dairy Products**. Do not drink cow's milk, in a glass, or have it in your coffee, in your baking, or on your cereal. Eliminate butter, all the cheeses like cheese from cows, goats and sheep, cottage cheese, yogurt, sour cream, and ice cream.[17,18] There are many dairy replacement products that are just as unhealthy as dairy, those made with soy protein isolates.[19] Avoid the vegan versions of cream cheese, sour cream, cheese slices, and ice creams.

- **Eggs**. Eliminate eggs and egg-containing products that are present in baked goods, and mayonnaise. This includes the vegan-style mayonnaise products, as they're packed with oils.[9-13]

- **Vegetable oils**. Eliminate all oils from your diet. Instead of sautéing your vegetables in oil, try a vegetable stock or plain water. You can sauté your mushrooms in water. If you watch carefully, you can even brown them in a non-stick pan. You will find them just as delicious without being smothered in greasy oil. You can make tasty fat-free salad dressings. You can also substitute apple sauce or bananas for vegetable oils in baking. Commercial crackers and baked goods like doughnuts and cookies are full of oil and refined flour and are not part of healthy eating. Cookies, chocolate, and candy bars are also full of trans fats, the worst kind of oil. All oils are fat that will end up in your fat cells.[9-13]

- **Refined flour and sugar**. Flours and sugar have had all their nutrient value taken out by over processing. Some of the most common flours are refined, such as white, wheat flour and white rice flour. When purchasing breads, pastas, or other flour-based products, look for those that are multi-grain or sprouted grain. Avoid refined sugar and sugar coated cereals. Dr. McDougall does allow you to sprinkle a bit of sugar on the surface of your food for simple pleasure. Don't worry, unless you eat large amounts of sugar, it won't make you fat.[20]

- **Odds and ends**. It's best to eliminate coffee, decaffeinated coffee and black teas, colas and pop, coconuts and any products made with soy protein isolates.[4,18] At first, reduce your caffeine consumption to no more than one cup daily, and then to one-half cup daily, before taking it out altogether. This will lessen symptoms of caffeine withdrawal, such as headache.

Exercise – It's the Extra Ingredient for a Better You!

To balance the road to optimal health, Dr. McDougall suggests you get some daily exercise. It is one of the cornerstones to regaining your health. Start with a ten minute walk every day and then in the second week, add five minutes to each walk. Every week add five more minutes until you have reached the minimum 45 minutes for your daily walk.[21]

This daily walk can add a wonderful sense of well-being to your life. Dr. McDougall stresses the importance of exercise. He says it helps you maintain a normal appetite, gives you energy, helps you sleep, improves circulation, digestion, blood pressure, blood sugar, and triglyceride levels, and the list goes on.[21] Dr. Neal Barnard wants you to know that regular physical activity, such as walking 45 minutes, four times per week, reduces the risk of developing dementia and Alzheimer's disease.[22]

If you are unable to walk, just stretching and moving your arms up over your head and rotating your ankles will be a good start. Do what you can do, but do it. Exercise is vital to better health and longevity.

Keep in mind that those who exercise experience a greater sense of self-esteem and improved mood, along with reduced anxiety and stress levels.[23] The main component of creating health is choosing a healthy eating plan which we have outlined here, but adding exercise completes the journey to perfect health.

So You Want to Lose Massive Amounts of Weight

Once you have mastered *The Starch Solution* program and have started to regain your health and lose some of your extra weight, you may find that your weight loss levels off, but you still have more weight to lose. It is not unusual to lose 20 to 50 pounds in the first year following *The Starch Solution* program with no extra effort, but you may still need to lose another 30 pounds or more. That is when you can switch to following the advice in Dr. McDougall's book, *The McDougall Program for Maximum Weight Loss*.[24] Once you have lost all the weight you wish to lose, go back to the regular program. This is what you will follow for the rest of your life. It will become your chosen lifestyle. You will never be sick, hungry, or fat again.

Dr. McDougall designed this weight loss program for people who are focused on one thing and one thing only, and that is getting rid of this unattractive, extra weight, once and for all, quickly and permanently. They are tired of being hungry and fat all the time. They want to look and feel great. The added bonus of this diet is regaining excellent health.[24]

As you settle into the program for seven days or so, and if you are following it 100 percent, you will realize that your body and appetite are content with the new types of foods you are eating. Weight is coming off and your health is improving all at the same time.[24] The biggest struggle with dieting is that to lose weight, you must go against your basic and most powerful instinct - your hunger drive. When you diet, by calorie restricting, you will be hungry all the time. It will be the return of that monster hunger drive that we mentioned earlier. Instead, by making healthy starches the center of your meals, and eating as much as you want of the right foods, you will be satisfied and happy and you won't feel deprived.

Most overweight and obese people have tried many different diets. If you are eating fats and animal proteins, your body is craving carbohydrates. Carbohydrates turn into glycogen in your body, which is the fuel your cells need for energy and good health.[20] If you are not getting enough carbohydrates, you will continue to crave them, continue to overeat and continue to feel dissatisfied. This feeling of being hungry all the time is your body attempting to find the carbohydrate it needs.[25]

Most of the diets that people are familiar with, like the Atkin's diet and the Paleo diet, are carbohydrate-deficient diets. McDougall's program does not work on that principle. In fact, it gives your body all the carbohydrates it needs while eliminating the fatty foods that the body doesn't need which, in turn, allows you to lose weight and get healthy at the same time.[4,24] The typical standard Western diet is four times as dense in calories as this program. High carbohydrate meals increase your energy and are much lower in calories. The added bonus: Unlike diets that are high in animal fats, it is unlikely you will ever feel sleepy after you eat.[24]

If you faithfully follow the program, Dr. McDougall assures you that you can anticipate losing anywhere from six to fifteen pounds each month. The more you weigh when you start the program, the more weight you can expect to lose in the first months. The results are going to be significant, and the weight loss is going to be permanent for overweight people who commit to this plan.[24]

If you are on your last 10 to 20 pounds and have reached a plateau, try increasing your exercise and modify your plate of food so you are taking in more green and yellow vegetables.[24] If your plateau continues, we encourage you to follow the recommendations in the next section.

Simple Changes for Maximum Weight Loss

You are going to continue following the dietary guidelines that have been outlined earlier in this chapter, but you are going to undertake some further restrictions while you are focused on losing the maximum amount of weight.

- Eliminate nuts, seeds, avocados, olives, soybean products like tofu, soy cheese and soy milk. These are plant foods that are high in fat. By not eating any fat during this restricted time, your body will dip into your fat stores to retrieve the fat it needs to operate optimally causing you to lose weight.[24]

- Eliminate anything made with flour. That means no bread, muffins, crackers, pasta, wraps, processed cereals, etc. Flour is a processed food that has been ground down into the tiniest particles. These particles are digested more readily in the small intestine, and are transferred into the bloodstream much more efficiently than larger particles. You get more calories to burn with these tiny particles of flour, and they end up slowing down weight loss.[24]

- Limit fruit to two servings per day. Eliminate fruit juices, and dried fruits as well as fruit puree.[24]

Other Good Ideas for Losing the Maximum Amount of Weight:

- Fill one-third to one-half of your plate with green and yellow vegetables. These will lower the caloric density of your entire meal because they have a quarter the number of calories as your starchy vegetable. These foods are packed with vitamins and minerals and trace nutrients.[24]

- Eat as many raw vegetables as you can as they cause you to lose more weight. Celery, carrots, broccoli, snow peas, bell peppers, and salad greens can all be eaten raw. Cooking breaks down the components of the carbohydrates making them more easily digestible and, therefore, higher in calories.[24]

A Few Words of Encouragement

Unlike most diets, when on this program, you can eat until you are satisfied with the foods previously listed. Interestingly, when you are full, you are less likely to lose control and stray off the program. With a tummy full of starchy carbohydrate foods that are oil-free, your appetite will be curbed and you can successfully regain your good looks and perfect weight. Everyone around you will be impressed with your seemingly disciplined lifestyle.[24]

You can have snacks and graze and have as many small meals as you would like, as long as you are eating from the allowed list of foods. If you are hungry, you can eat and feel satisfied. Have some "go to" starches prepared for when you get hungry.[24] For example, you could have a bowl of cooked steel cut oats available for a late-night snack which you smother in grapes or berries. It is something you could look forward to in the evenings and find completely satisfying.

It is helpful to know you don't have to have a great variety of food on this program. You can eat hot oatmeal for breakfast, rice for lunch, and potatoes for dinner, every day. These foods provide the foundation to which you can add a green or yellow vegetable, or one of your two allowed fruits. This is more than enough nutritional content to keep you healthy and lose weight steadily. It is not necessary to prepare difficult recipes. In fact, you are more likely to experience success in the first few weeks if you make simple, hearty meals.

Chapter Five
Amy

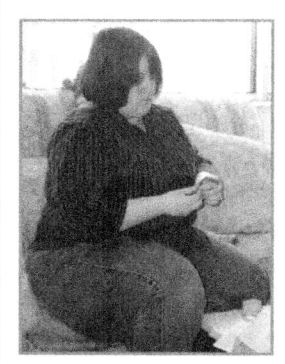

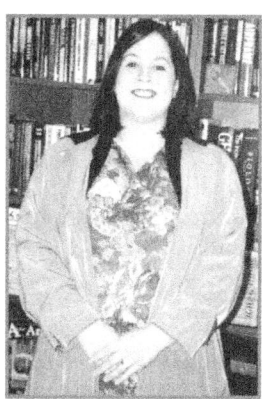

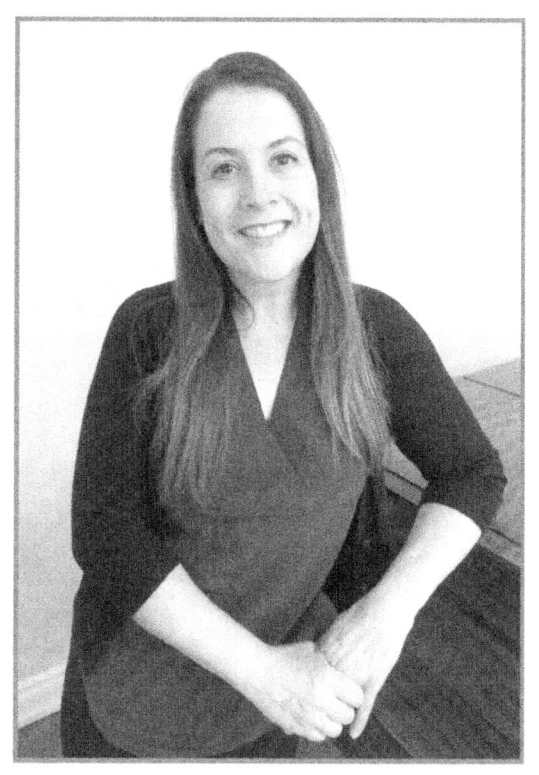

Amy had a weight problem her whole life. She tried every diet there is, with no long term success. Other health issues, like diabetes and arthritis were looming. Then, Amy discovered Dr. McDougall, and has since lost more than 110 pounds. In this interview, she shares her tools of success to get thin and healthy forever.

**Toronto Starch Solution Meetup Group
Group Toronto Starch Solution Meetup**

Chapter Five - Amy's Interview

Amy, please share with us some background information about your life, your job, and your family.

I have been overweight or obese for most of my life. Even in my early teens I could be described as thick. I distinctly remember being very preoccupied with my weight from a very young age. As a teenager, I was slightly overweight and did manage one summer to diet my way down to a normal size. It required a very low calorie diet of 800 calories a day and cycling 15 kilometres a day (along a tranquil residential stretch of road, Spruce Avenue from Guelph Line to Burloak Drive in Burlington). But I couldn't maintain this level of calories and I didn't maintain this level of exercise. The weight crept back up and I was over 200 pounds by the time I was 19 years old. My early twenties were spent jumping from one popular diet to the next with limited success. Twenty pounds down, twenty-five pounds up. Two steps forward, three steps back.

In my mid-twenties, I decided to go the ultra-low calorie route that had worked in my teens. My mom and sister and I all went to a popular diet clinic where you were weighed three times a week and given Vitamin B shots while severely limiting calories and fat. We all lost weight. I lost more than 70 pounds in the course of 6 months. The day I stopped going to the clinic was the day I started to gain the weight back. During that time, I met and married my husband, bought a house, started my career, and got busy with living my life. We soon started a family.

Could you please tell us about your journey to Dr. McDougall. When did you find him? How has the Starch Solution Program impacted your life?

In 2005, after the birth of my third child, the health consequences of being obese began to catch up with me and I was not yet 31 years old. That year, my BMI topped out at an all-time high of 45; I was a five foot and half an inch tall, female, weighing in at 237 pounds. That equates to the highest level of obesity standardly measured: Class 3 morbid obesity. The year prior, I had my gallbladder removed, and the surgeon had prescribed me statins. Additionally, my blood pressure began to creep up and my back and knees and hips and fingers were always sore and stiff.

That year, I happened upon the book, *Eat to Live* by Dr. Joel Fuhrman. To say I happened upon it is a little disingenuous. Like many chronic dieters, not only did I live on an intermittent stream of junk food, I also consumed a constant stream of pop science diet literature. When I read this book, I tried to follow the plan and failed. I didn't think anything of it; just another diet book. The seeds of truth in that book did not sprout. I continued to read other books from the likes of Dr. Mark Hyman, and a variety of low carb books. That was still my fall-back diet when I wanted a few pounds off quickly. I had no idea at the time that most of that weight loss was only water, or that I was potentially harming myself.

In the following year, I read a book my local library had featured called *The Great Starvation Experiment* by historian Todd Tucker. It looked like an interesting account about the history of conscientious objectors during World War II, just something fun to read, not diet related. These men were involved in an experiment that systematically starved them in order for the US government to potentially learn about the best way to help the starving people of Europe postwar. The experiments were run by Dr. Ancel Keyes, creator of the K-ration and researcher/author of *The Seven Countries Study*. This book serendipitously led me back in the right direction. It led me to looking up caloric restriction, which led me to reading about the historic diet of the Okinawans, which led me to Dr. T. Colin Campbell's book, *The China Study*, which led me to Dr. McDougall.

All of the information began to coalesce. I began to realize how importantly connected chronic disease and diet were. I read about the increase in chronic disease rates when eastern populations stopped eating traditional foods. Problems started when they took up a more Western diet, heavier in refined foods and animal-based products, especially dairy.

However, this doesn't mean I was able to just take this information and run with it. Oh, if only! It took many more years of experimenting with how close to the guidelines I needed to be in order to get results. I began a cycle of yo-yo dieting, going on and off the program. By 2010, I was exasperated with myself. Why wasn't I able to follow these guidelines? By now, I had found Dr. McDougall's website and was delving more deeply into the world of whole food plant-based eating. I had reached a point where I knew there was no need to keep looking for the Holy Grail of diets, I had found it. I just needed to figure out how to stay on it!

As it happens, I had a good year following the plan and was excited to find out that I was pregnant. My husband and I had wanted another child and had been trying to get pregnant since the last birth in 2005. I attribute it to the diet. The pregnancy was not an easy one, I was still quite obese and had developed gestational diabetes in the second trimester. I received a prescription for insulin, which I used only when I was having trouble eating by the McDougall program guidelines. When I ate what was recommended, I was able to manage the diabetes with the dietary changes alone. Through the course of that year and pregnancy, I lost 40 pounds and delivered a healthy baby in 2011. Then I went back to eating the way I had always eaten and gained much of the weight back. When would I ever learn?

So, I kept reading. Next up was Dr. McDougall's book, *The Starch Solution*. At the time, what kept bringing me back to Dr. McDougall, specifically (versus the many other quality plant-based practitioners in this sphere), was his passion and integrity. Like all of us, he needed to make a living and support his family, but he also felt it necessary to share all of the information he was gathering and applying with his patients to anyone who would read it for free online. He didn't want anyone to not have access to how to live a healthy life, following scientific best practices, if they came looking for it. I really appreciated that. Through his website, I learned about the book *The Pleasure Trap* by psychologist Dr. Doug Lisle and chiropractor Dr. Alan Goldhamer. This was the piece of information I had been missing.

I struggle with addictive tendencies. I was a moderate to heavy smoker from my mid-teens until my first pregnancy. I also drank more than I am proud to admit during my twenties. I used both of these things to calm my internal maelstrom. I used food in much the same way, and still have the tendency to do that. Understanding that I self-medicate with a variety of addictive and quasi-addictive items was not enough to keep me from doing it. It also wasn't enough to keep me from despairing about why I couldn't stop doing it. Reading, *The Pleasure Trap* was what it took. That book was instrumental in changing my understanding about why I was continually struggling to eat a very healthy diet, when I knew it was the best plan for my health and weight loss. I read about Dr. Lisle's concept, the motivational triad, hyper-palatable foods, and the toxic food environment. I came away realizing there wasn't anything wrong with me. All of those years of anguishing that if I could only temper my appetite, or use my willpower just a bit longer, were such a waste of energy and emotion. I was doing what I was designed to do, and simply needed to adjust my environment. I realized that's what I had to do in order to have success, because I couldn't change my personality or genetics.

Alas, even this new understanding didn't bring me instant weight loss and success. I struggled in a household that ate many different ways, and thus, I was constantly put in temptation's path. I struggled with having to explain my different way of eating to people who looked at me in disbelief. I didn't look like one should if they were eating a healthy diet. I struggled to do this alone, all by myself, without someone to talk to about it and share the good and bad days. However, once you understand there are best practices to follow, and that the research literature supports this, there is no turning back. I couldn't just stop trying because it was difficult, because I knew better.

I continued to restart the plan each and every day. I continued to talk about it with my family, even if I wasn't a shining example of success. By 2014, I had gained back what little weight I had lost during my last pregnancy. I know that doesn't sound right, but you read it correctly. That year, my doctor tested me for two different autoimmune diseases based on symptoms. I knew that both of these diseases were highly manageable, and even reversible, by following an oil-free plant-based diet. Any time I had to get blood work done, I would follow the guidelines perfectly and my blood work would turn out just fine. I knew I was complicating things. I also knew I was starting to get sick and needed to improve my compliance track record.

Then life threw us for another loop. My mom got sick. She didn't just get a little sick, she got a lot sick. She was diagnosed with breast cancer and Parkinson's disease within a few months of each other. As she went through conventional cancer treatment, I pushed a bit harder about the dietary changes I had been trying to make and how they may help her. I wasn't always eloquent and I wasn't always tactful. I learned a lot about how not to persuade someone to your cause. I guess you could say I was a bit pushy. My mom asked me to show her some results, and then she would consider listening.

I started back at it, seriously, at the end of 2014. By the spring of 2015, only four months later, I had dropped 25 pounds. I was feeling encouraged and my family seemed to be listening and supporting me more. Mom was now officially in remission and life was settling down into a peaceful interlude. Then, the music stopped and there was one less chair to sit on. Mom called one morning to let me and my siblings know that something unusual had been seen on an X-ray, and that she was going to have additional tests. There was a chance that her cancer may have returned. We were devastated by this news.

During that call, I told her about the 10-day live in program offered by the McDougall Wellness Center. There were many success stories, including people that had apparently cured their cancer by following this diet. I sent my mom the story of Ruth Heidrich, who was an early patient of Dr. McDougall's and had success treating her late stage breast cancer that had spread to her lungs. Mom agreed to attend the program, and I began to try and figure out how I was going to swing going away for ten days. My mom decided to make it a family health vacation, and my dad and siblings joined us and attended the program.

We all went in June of 2015 to Santa Rosa, California. We got to see the whole crew including Dr. McDougall, and Jeff Novick, the program's registered dietitian. Heather McDougall, who is Dr. McDougall's daughter, runs the clinic. Mary McDougall, Dr. McDougall's wife, developed all of the delicious recipes. She provides support on how to grocery shop and eat out. There were a number of different chefs: Cathy Fisher, Chef Bravo, and Jill Nussinow, *The Vegan Under Pressure* cook book author, and, of course, Dr. Lisle, the staff psychologist. They all did presentations. Michelle and Tiffany ensured everything ran smoothly behind the scenes. It's a pretty fantastic experience that I recommend to anyone who will listen.

This vacation was an inflection point for me. I figured out quite quickly that I hadn't been eating large enough meals to stay satisfied, and that I thrived on meeting others also trying to figure out how to eat this way consistently in our toxic food environment. Since then, I have slowly but surely continued to lose weight. I am down over 100 pounds now. I think that's pretty amazing. I am so proud of myself.

It hasn't been without struggles. I still fall into the pleasure trap quite often, but I now have strategies to get back on track quickly before things get out of hand. The post program support has been wonderful. Jeff Novick continues to work with each of us, and he's always available to answer our questions – often within minutes. He has a forum on the McDougall website that may be my most visited spot for knowledge and inspiration. I am in awe of his ability to refer to any number of resources when responding to questions off the top of his head. He is a true expert in his field.

I still have a way to go, but I feel confident that I will get there. My obesity needs to be managed like a disease and the treatment is the proper natural diet we evolved to eat. As long as I continue the treatment, my disease will stay in remission. It's that simple. Now, as we have seen, staying the course has been difficult for me. Simple does not mean easy. But like a musician learning to play the piano, or an athlete learning to excel in her sport, it just takes practice, lots and lots of practice. I am practicing how to navigate each and every situation I find myself in. I don't always do well the first time, but you can bet I will have a plan for the next time. One other thing that I have learned is that weight loss takes way more time than you think it will. To comfortably eat under your hunger drive means not going too low on the calories. You can expect only up to one pound a week of weight loss. I would be thrilled with more, but don't expect it.

Here are some of the strategies that I use to get through each day. I didn't invent any of these techniques. They are from Jeff Novick, Dr. McDougall, Dr. Lisle and some of the longtime McDougallers who post so much helpful information on the McDougall website:

1) Be prepared. Always have food made and ready to be eaten. Pre-cook potatoes and rice. Chop vegetables and fruit. Make soups and stews and freeze them in individual portions.

2) Pre-eat before socializing. If you are going out and don't know if you will have access to healthy food, eat before you go. That will buy you time and let you enjoy your outing.

3) Bring food with you wherever you go. It's always a good idea to travel with a meal. Again, just to keep yourself from being tempted in case you allowed yourself to get too hungry.

4) Don't eat after your evening meal. Night time snacking can stall weight loss and lead to bingeing in those who are susceptible (me!). I sip sparkling water or have tea to get through the evenings.

5) Eat your meal in order of calorie density. Start with soup and/or salad, follow with vegetables and fruit and then eat your starch. You will fill up on less calories.

6) Walk four to five times a week. It feels good.

7) Join support groups online, create support groups in real life. Having people to talk to about this most important human activity (eating) is so important. As you have already read, the ladies here in Toronto started a starch-based potluck group, and boy, has it grown!

It sounds like this changed your life in a big way.

Definitely. I am happy! I am so very happy. When you are very, very, obese, not only is it physically draining, it is mentally draining. Getting through everyday life is difficult. I couldn't make any long-term plans because I didn't see a future. I didn't have the energy to even try to see one. It, at times, felt like a sad, small life. Struggling to do all of the things you are responsible for to the best of your ability, knowing that you are not doing a great job at anything because you are just so physically drained. Another thing that has changed is the subtle cues from people around me. An obese person wears their vice, unlike other perceived "moral failings" that can be hidden from sight. You are a walking billboard for what people think of as character flaws. Sloth and gluttony come to mind. I was not blind to the subtle disgust, or to being treated like I was invisible. Men and women both do this. I too am guilty of judging others by their appearance. I work very hard to correct this tendency because we don't know what path someone has been on before it crosses our own.

What would you say have been your biggest obstacles or difficulties?

The concept Dr. Lisle presents, called the pleasure trap, is where I still consistently have issues. The ease of which someone is able to adopt these types of dietary changes will depend upon your personality. Dr. Lisle explains the Factor Five or Big Five Plus One personality assessment, and how your individual personality affects dietary compliance in a lecture on his website called *The Perfect Personality*. All of our personality characteristics fall on a continuum in five different areas: introversion/extroversion, conscientiousness/openness to experience, agreeability/disagreeability and excitability. There are a few people who have the perfect personality to succeed on this diet easily. They aren't affected by sugar, salt and oil. They will read the information and say, "This is great information," and change their diet the next day. They will eat this way every day for the rest of their lives, like Dr. Alan Goldhamer or Chef AJ, according to Dr. Lisle. But some people are going to struggle based on those personality parameters. I am one of those people. I struggle every single day and it doesn't ever go away. I can only eat one or two too salty or too sweet things and then I will feel a little itch in the back of my head saying, "Have more, eat more." That is a constant battle for me.

The McDougall Maximum Weight-loss Program seems to be the best version of the program for someone like me. When you are slipping up every day you are reinforcing a certain neural pathway, and you need to let that degrade a bit so it doesn't have such a pull on you. People who are highly addictive don't think it can be done, because it is so hard to apply the guidelines for a long enough period of time to see the results. Once you do, you realize you can be free of this addictive behaviour. It does become easier, until you slip up again. That has been my hardest battle. I continue to read. I have re-read *The Pleasure Trap* and other books on why we do things the way we do them, to glean a little more understanding of my limitations when it comes to hyper-palatable foods. These foods are ones that don't exist in nature, and are very high in stimulants like sugar, salt, fat, and caffeine.

What kinds of things do you like to eat?

For myself, I have learned to love simple foods. But that has evolved over time. My lunch and evening meal consists of a fruit, a starch, such as brown rice or potatoes, a bean soup or stew, and some raw or steamed vegetables. There are so many great recipes, blogs and websites available now. Vegetarian awareness has exploded, as Jeff Novick, RD, had said at the program in 2015. He said the next big thing is going to be the vegan diet but not to be fooled. It is a vegan junk food diet that's going to be offered. Industry is going to swoop in because this is the next big money-making food trend, much like the low-fat movement in the 80s with Snackwells and Fig Newtons. He is right. From 2005 until now, it is like night and day with regards to the recipes you can find online. I am thankful because a small percentage of them are oil-free, so we have many choices.

I am not a creative cook. I am not going to experiment or develop a recipe. That's not me. I will follow a recipe word for word and make it. Though I am thankful for the spotlight being shone on the health benefits of a plant-based diet, I am concerned much of the benefit will not make it to mainstream eating due to a misapplication of the principles. It has the potential to be the 1980s again where people became discouraged because they thought they were eating a healthier low-fat diet, but evidence indicates they were not. They threw out the baby with the bathwater on that concept.

Where does your support come from?

So many places. It took a long time to figure that out. My husband is my number one champion. My extended family and friends have taken up my cause as their own, and will always ensure that I am able to socialize with them. They always provide something acceptable for me to eat. That everyone has rallied around me brings a big smile to my face and an even bigger feeling of gratitude. Once I made this my lifestyle, and not my current diet, and everyone saw how much better I was feeling and looking, they all wanted to help me stay the course. The people in my life had front row seats to my frustrating and sometimes disheartening struggle to be well. No one wants to tempt me back down that path.

You can feel so alone when you are changing the way you are eating. You are doing something so different from most people. Add to that some limiting health complications and low self-esteem due to consistently failing to achieve a goal you so desperately desire. That's the perfect recipe for depression. I, personally, belong to a support group that includes just the people who I attended the 10-day McDougall program with. It is a small group, and we bonded by experiencing the program together, graduating, and then going back to our individual lives. They are my plant-based family. Though we live far apart, they are in my thoughts and we check in with each other frequently. I also rely quite heavily on the McDougall discussion forums at mcdougall.com. It is a very large group with a variety of backgrounds, interests, and temperaments. There is always something new to read and comment on. I began facilitating the Maximum Weight Loss (MWL) weigh-in thread in November of 2016. It has given me the opportunity to interact with many people new to this lifestyle, and to help guide them through the information available to them on the website. Everyone needs something just a little different, and I'm happy to help them find those resources.

With so much online support, I also realized that I needed some in-person support. I was new to the area and decided that I would join the local vegetarian association. At the same time, by chance, some of the ladies you may have already read about here, were reaching out to members of the McDougall forum who lived in Toronto. They were looking for in-person support too and that's how the Toronto Starch Solution Meetup group was born.

Do you have any advice for beginners?

This is a good question. In my mind, the person I am advising is a beginner who is obese, who is struggling with the same addiction-like issues that I struggle with. That is who I would identify with. That would be the kind of beginner I am speaking to. To them I would say, realize that this will take longer than you think to get right, but it is so worthwhile to keep trying. Additionally, and not to sound repetitive, but this is so important, don't internalize your obesity and inability to diet your way out of it as a personal failing or a character flaw. You can take away the mental anguish surrounding your self-image by realizing the deck truly is stacked against you in this particular arena. What you have been experiencing is merely an application problem. So, first off, read one of the many plant-based no-oil diet programs available. I'm partial to Dr. McDougall, as you may have guessed. Secondly, read *The Pleasure Trap*, twice! Those were the two most helpful things for me.

Let's talk about your future plans. How do you see yourself impacting the world with this new information?

I definitely have that passion. I am still up in the air a little bit as to where I can best be of service to others. John McDougall, Neal Barnard and many of the other "vegan doctors" have decided to try and change the world. Big picture stuff. They are writing bills for government change and suing the government, writing books and giving seminars. Alternately, Jeff Novick once wrote that this is not his focus, and I identify with his approach a little bit more. Jeff said he is going to work his hardest helping people who come looking for the help. He is going to work his hardest for those already searching and in need of the best answer. He recognized that this was going to be something like 0.1% of the population. If he is able to help them achieve better health, he would feel highly satisfied with his life's work. He is not out to fight the people not looking for this help. I think that is the group that I wish to focus on as well. I believe, however, both types of approaches are necessary to bring about large scale change, and have a big effect on public health and the epidemic of chronic disease and obesity we are experiencing globally.

We needed to start as a grassroots type movement, with people learning from the experience of the ones they know who have benefited, learning from the professionals who had to work outside of the medical system but had been trained within it. These people will then begin to ask for change in the government regulations and policies surrounding food, nutrition, and industry influence. If enough people begin to ask for changes, politicians will begin to ask for them as well. We need enough experts advising the policy makers and enough citizens demanding changes of their governments for this to work. We are fighting human nature here.

What's your opinion on animal rights and the impact of an animal-based diet on the environment?

I came to the whole food plant-based eating world for health reasons, but when you read enough you can't help but begin to understand the negative environmental impact of large-scale livestock farming. So much land and water is used for feeding these animals, land and water that could be better allocated to growing grain crops for human consumption. This leads one to also consider the inhumane treatment of these animals when they become commodities for consumption versus living beings. We have created a nice tidy system where our food comes in packages and boxes in clean, well-lit stores. We don't have to see the process of how a pig becomes a pork chop or bacon or a hot dog. Thus, we don't tend to think about it, and we don't tend to question it. That is how companies involved in this type of work want it. That is how factory farms came to be. I can't imagine getting to the place we are now if there had been more transparency. All of us have compassion. We are just so far removed from our food production that we have no idea what it has become, and slowly, checks and balances were removed and lines were crossed one tiny step at a time for the sake of efficiency and the bottom line.

The longer you stay in this space for health you can't help but become aware of the other issues. Some people enter as an ethical vegan and gain better health as an unforeseen benefit. Others come to cure a disease and begin to realize how what they eat affects the environment. It just all makes sense. The most health promoting diet, is also the most environmentally friendly diet, is also the most ethical diet. What a glorious Venn diagram we could draw here. Here is my purse. This is a vegan purse. I never would have thought about that before. I am making different choices now. Do I get rid of my car because it has a leather interior? Not yet. Will I purchase leather interior in the future? Possibly not. Making all these little choices can have a big impact. We can make big changes by voting with our dollars, by supporting companies whose values are in tune with our own. Some of us will change all at once and others, like me, just gently move in that direction whenever I am faced with a choice that I had previously not considered very deeply.

Do you see yourself changing the world?

I see myself changing my world. I will be happy if my friends and family choose to learn a little bit more. That is my primary goal. If that ripples over into a larger group I would be thrilled. One change I would love to see is a copy of PCRM's (Physicians Committee for Responsible Medicine) Nutrition Guide for Clinicians in every doctor's office and dietitian's clinic at the hospital. To have dietary change presented as an equally or more effective treatment to conventional treatments for heart disease, diabetes, lupus, MS and many, many other conditions, could go a long way in giving patients a truly informed choice on how to best manage their disease. If a patient chooses a conventional surgical or pharmacological treatment, so be it. I accept that, but I think many people would give this a shot if they knew its efficacy.

John McDougall has taken it a step farther than that with this latest bill he is working on. He is mandating that doctors have to legally tell their patients that the heart medicine won't prolong their life, and the heart procedure is not going to save their life either but a plant-based diet will. With diabetics it is the same thing, as it gives people the chance to make an informed decision. That is what he put forward to Congress.

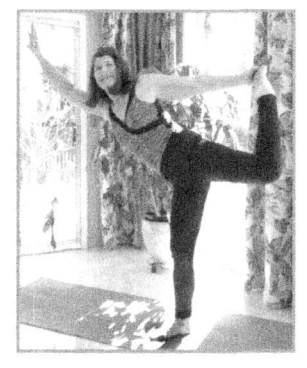

Chapter Six
Diane

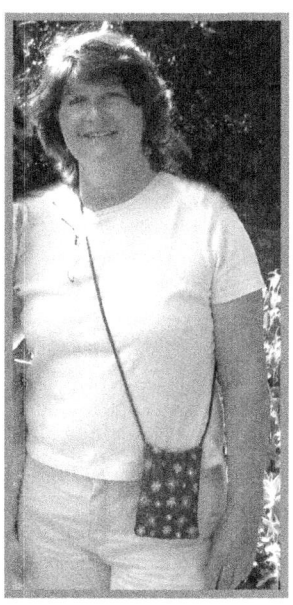

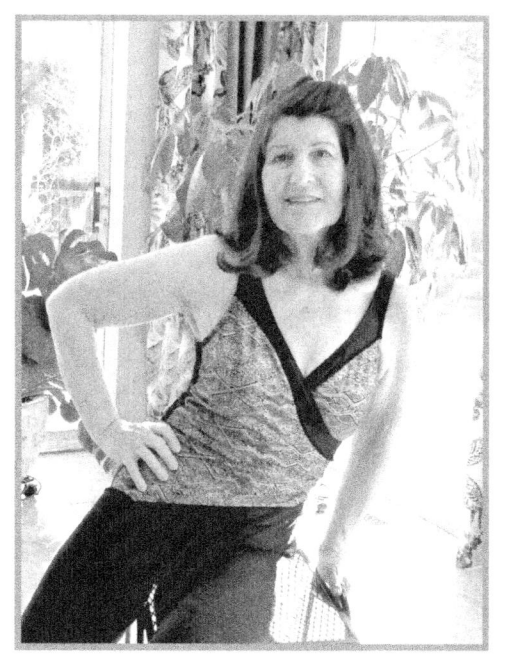

Diane knew she was in deep trouble. After having one of her hips replaced, many of her other joints were now becoming progressively swollen, painful and damaged with arthritis. Read about her journey back to vibrant health with a bonus weight loss of 53 pounds, all thanks to Dr. McDougall. Now she is active in hiking, yoga, and living completely pain free.

Toronto Starch Solution Meetup Group
Group Toronto Starch Solution Meetup

Chapter Six - Diane's Interview

Diane, tell us about your background, marital status, children, that sort of thing.

I was a professional photographer and worked at the Art Gallery of Ontario as their staff photographer. I got married and pregnant. I decided to quit my job, stay home with the two kids and just work on weekends shooting weddings. When my kids were young, I got divorced. At that point, I started buying income real estate. I bought and sold houses. Now, I'm retired and I am living with my father in the west end of Toronto.

Tell us your story in relation to *The Starch Solution* Program.

I ate the standard Western diet with meat, dairy, and a few fruits and veggies. I ate lots of junk food like cookies and chocolate bars my whole life. I didn't eat chips or drink pop. I was under the impression that I was eating healthy. When I was 52 years old, I was living in the beaches of Toronto. I woke up one morning and my hip was really sore. I thought I must have pulled it. I did practice yoga at the time and was going three times a week. This hip was really sore and I was hobbling around. I kept thinking that it will get better, but it never did. I ended up having to quit my yoga practice. That was so disappointing.

The dog wasn't too happy either that I couldn't walk anymore. What I could do was ride my bike. So, the dog learned to run alongside the bike. I learned how to live with a sore hip. I just figured I was getting old.

Then, years passed. It's really incredible how the years passed, and I just adapted to not being able to walk very far. I got lots of exercise by riding around the neighbourhood on my bike. Finally, I began to realize I was making a huge compromise in my lifestyle by not being able to walk. That's when I saw my doctor. She took x-rays, and informed me that the cartilage was completely gone from my right hip joint and that I was a candidate for a hip replacement. By this time, I was 58 years old. She wasn't sure what kind of arthritis had caused this kind of damage.

I went to a surgeon who was a hip specialist. In Ontario, you have to wait a year for your free surgery, which is covered under our public healthcare system. It turned out that I was allergic to some common metals, so the surgeon arranged for me to get a special titanium hip joint. Then, I had the surgery.

As an incentive to recover quickly, I booked a two-week European cruise that would start three months after having the surgery. That was the perfect goal to get me back on my feet fast and get walking. I intended to do a lot of walking on my trip. My strategy worked. I had a wonderful time in Europe and was able to walk without pain. I am grateful for my new titanium hip joint and the amazing team of trained specialists who performed the operation.

It was October when I got back from the cruise and the cold weather was setting in. Then, something strange was happening. With the onset of the cool, damp weather, my other hip started hurting. Both my knees were swollen and sore. My back was killing me and my fingers were as big as bananas. The arthritis was hitting like gang busters. I knew I was in real trouble and I was scared.

I arranged to see an arthritis specialist. This specialist told me there is no cure for arthritis. He painted a grim picture of what my future entailed. He prescribed a heavy-duty painkiller and an anti-inflammatory drug with nasty side effects like bleeding from your rectum. He wanted me to go to a six-week government funded program called "How to Live with Arthritis".

This same thing happened to my mother. She was shrivelled, bent and swollen with arthritis. She was in a wheelchair for the last ten years of her life. She had her knee joints replaced when she was in her early sixties, but it was her deteriorated back bone that was the biggest problem. They put her on a risky painkiller called Celebrex. It is one of those drugs with nasty side effects like permanent diarrhea and a high increased risk of heart attack or stroke. She was in so much pain, she had no choice but to take the drug, just to have any sort of quality of life.

Mom also endured Alzheimer's and it was just the saddest thing to see her decline. She died at age 86 from a stroke probably caused by the Celebrex. Those last ten years of her life were tough. I knew I was heading down the same road as my mom. I had my first hip replacement at the age of 59. My knees were inflamed. My other hip was inflamed. My back was inflamed, and my fingers were inflamed. And to top it off, I couldn't find the car keys, and words were slipping out of my memory.

At this point, I didn't know what I was going to do. I knew I just had to find what was causing all this. I knew that something was causing this. I just had to find out what it was. I was determined I was going to get to a solution. I was resolute that I was not going to go down the same road as my poor mother.

I started researching on the internet and I googled "cure for arthritis". Guess who pops up? Dr. John McDougall pops up! He has hundreds of YouTube videos available, so I listened to that first lecture called, *The Starch Solution*. Then, I listened to practically every one of his lectures. I must have listened to him for a hundred hours. And of course, other people's lectures came up at the same time such as those of Dr. Caldwell Esselstyn, Dr. T. Colin Campbell, Dr. Neal Barnard, and Dr. Michael Greger. I listened to them all. All these amazing doctors are saying one thing. You can cure incurable diseases, like heart disease, diabetes, some cancers and arthritis with a whole food, plant-based, no-oil diet. I started considering what they were saying, maybe it was the food I was eating that was inflaming my joints and affecting my memory.

I made the decision that I was going to try this, to dive right in 100% for three months. I'm going to see if there's an improvement in my arthritis. I am going to follow Dr. John McDougall's whole food, starch-based, no-oil diet. I downloaded his 10-day program off his website, and bought two of his books, as well as the movie *Forks Over Knives*. I love that movie. Every time I need to get inspired, I watch that movie. It's now available on Netflix.

After I had made my decision, I sat down with my family. I live with my father, my nephew and his wife. I made the announcement that I was not going to eat any animal-based foods for three months, and I was going to see if I could cure my arthritis. My nephew, in disbelief, reacted, "Well, I'm not doing it! I'm not giving up meat!" And I said, "You can eat whatever you want. This is what I'm doing. But I want you to know that the food is going to change for me, and I'm going to stick to it."

I started the program. I started with John McDougall's recipes from his website. I started eating only porridge, rice, potatoes, beans, vegetables, and fruit. Well, after one week, my banana fingers were right back to normal. My knees were back to normal. My back didn't hurt anymore. My other hip was fine. The inflammation was completely gone. The red-hot pain everywhere had stopped. I was thrilled, of course, but I also found it hard to believe. That was in one week, seven days. I am not exaggerating! It was like a miracle, and it was so simple! All I had to do was cut out the meat, the dairy, the eggs, the fish, the oil, and the junk food, and I was cured.

A lot has changed since then. That was four years ago when I started. I have never looked back. I have never touched meat again. I haven't had a taste of meat in four years, which is great. I have lost my appetite for it. The thought of it makes me sick. It repulses me. I don't want to have anything to do with it.

I haven't had to take a painkiller in four years. I used to pop Ibuprofen like candy, four times a day for the arthritic pain. Dr. McDougall explains that these over-the-counter painkillers will actually make your arthritis worse in the long run.

For the first year, I was stoic on *The Starch Solution* program. I was just perfect. I never veered off. Dr. McDougall would have been impressed with me. I was too terrified of getting my arthritis back. You couldn't get me to eat anything that wasn't on the program. My arthritis was gone and I had lost 20 pounds without even trying to.

Then, the second year came along and I relaxed a bit. I guess I wanted to see what I could get away with, without getting inflammation. I started trying a bit of cheese, cookies, and chocolate. I found out my arthritis does flare up when I indulge in the occasional dairy product or oily treat. If I go out for dinner with friends and eat the pasta with cheese, there are consequences. When I eat cheese, a finger or a knee will swell up the next day. When I get back on the program, the inflammation will go away.

In that first year, I lost 20 pounds, just by following Dr. McDougall's *The Starch Solution* program. At the end of February, 2016, I decided I wanted to get rid of this last bit of weight. I still had another 30 lbs to lose to get down to where I really wanted to be. I got out the book, *McDougall's Program for Maximum Weight Loss*, and decided to follow that program, which is a stricter version of *The Starch Solution*.

You are not to eat anything that is made from refined flours like bread, bagels, or pasta. You can still have whole grains like oatmeal, or brown rice. As per the program, I stopped eating nuts and seeds which I was enjoying on my morning oatmeal and I stopped my tablespoon of ground flaxseed as well. I cut out the occasional avocado and tofu.

I decided I was going to do this for three months. On my computer, I set up a chart. I had a place where I could track what I ate, how I exercised, and what my challenges were for the day. In red, I highlighted anything I ate that was not on the program. Sometimes you want to have a little spaghetti with some marinara sauce on it. This really isn't bad food, except it's made of ground flour which isn't the best choice for efficient weight loss.

I set a three-month goal. I thought, I can do this for three months, and then, I can go back to the regular Starch Solution lifestyle. At lunch, I normally like a multigrain wrap with oil-free hummus, loaded with greens and raw vegetables. I changed to a plate of whole grain rice with a salad instead of my wrap. Oh, that was the hardest part, giving up that wrap.

My goal was to lose 12 pounds. I ended up losing 16 pounds in that three-month period, which was just amazing. I could never lose weight so easily in my entire adult life! My BMI is now 24.4. I haven't been this thin for 35 years! I still have another 16 pounds to go to get to my ultimate goal weight, but I'll tackle this last 16 pounds when I am hibernating in the winter months to come.

I live with my father and I cook for him. I make enough starch for both of us, either rice, beans or potatoes and then steamed veggies. I make him his small portion of meat, if he wants it. His potatoes always have a pat of butter on them, mine don't. Often, he gets a hummus veggie wrap for lunch. He is up to three or four vegan dinners per week now. He won't give up his cup of cow's milk each day. He has oatmeal every morning and lots of fruits and vegetables. The guy is 93 years old with a perfect brain and perfectly healthy body. I know I have added years onto his life, in the last four years, with this way of eating.

I live pain-free now with full use and range of all my limbs. My arthritis is in full remission, as long as I follow *The Starch Solution* plan. If I had listened to that medical professional, the arthritis specialist, I never would have been experiencing this kind of health ever again. I would probably be waiting in line for another hip replacement by now. The internet is such a powerful research tool, right at your fingertips, right in your own home. You have to get it into your head that you are the sole person responsible for your own health.

I am lucky that I never put much value on what the mainstream doctors say. I think they are operating on a very narrow bandwidth. They are limited to how they can treat chronic diseases by the Medical Association's rules and regulations. They treat chronic diseases with pharmaceuticals only.

A lot of people believe that whatever doctors say must be the best and only way for them to proceed. The doctors are educated with medical degrees so they must know. You assume that doctors are up to date with the latest medical research. They are not.

Our medical system is advanced when it comes to emergencies like broken bones, car accidents, acute infections, and hip replacements, but what they aren't good at is treating chronic conditions like heart disease, high blood pressure, arthritis, or diabetes. I've learned that the usual treatment for these ailments is a string of expensive drugs with nasty side effects that, in many cases, actually do not prolong your life expectancy. They treat the symptoms of the disease with drugs, but don't know what is actually causing the problem in the first place.

As Dr. McDougall and his colleagues have discovered, it is the food, the standard Western diet that is causing most of these chronic diseases. The big killers are heart disease, diabetes and cancer, and they are all curable with food. It is the meat, dairy, and junk food that is making you sick. You have to change the types of food you are eating to get well again. You are injuring yourself three times a day, at breakfast, at lunch, and at dinner with bad food choices like meat, dairy, and oils.

The internet virtually saved my life. It enabled me to find Dr. McDougall. My arthritis is gone and I have added thirty years of pain-free, active living onto my life by taking charge of my own health. I won't be crippled with arthritis or be unable to recognize my loved ones because of Alzheimer's in this lifetime. It was the food that was making me sick. It was the meat, dairy products, and junk food.

The arthritis specialist told me there is no cure for my arthritis. He wanted to put me on a dicey pain medicine and a dangerous anti-inflammatory. He was sending me to a government-funded course on how to live with arthritis! Had I followed his advice, I would have been doomed to a life of disability, pain, and misery. Why is this doctor not informed? He is revered as an expert in his medical field and yet he doesn't know about the most effective and only cure available, which is a simple plant-based diet. The evidence is published in peer-reviewed medical journals. Is this not absurd?

Doctors, in positions of authority, armed with medical credentials, are doing such a disservice to hundreds of thousands of people who are in life-threatening situations. The tragedy is they are not learning about nutrition in medical school and using it as a powerful tool to actually help people to get well. This is such a large scale oversight. It is time for our medical system to change its focus from treating illness with drugs, to treating illness with food instead.

My advice to you is to take control of your own health! The information is on the internet, right at your fingertips. I saved my own life. I control what foods go in my body. I control the exercise I do daily. I control how interactive I am with my friends and family. I control how much sleep I get. I control the amount of laughter I create.

If you give your body the right food it will heal itself. Dr. McDougall and his colleagues have proven this beyond a shadow of doubt. Nine out of ten life-threatening chronic diseases are caused by eating meat, dairy, eggs and fish, and oils. It is easy to change your diet and lifestyle. It is hard to die like my mother did.

Who else has inspired you?

Well, Dr. McDougall is the top dog for sure! Dr. Neal Barnard, he has been a huge inspiration for me because my mother had Alzheimer's and the fact that there is an Alzheimer's gene that you definitely do not want to turn on. He has a video on YouTube called *Power Foods for Your Brain*, which is about how to prevent Alzheimer's and dementia.

I was so inspired by that talk, and I now know I won't be going down the Alzheimer's road either. I did a lot of damage to my brain in 60 years of eating crummy food. My memory wasn't that great but it has improved. Before changing my diet, I couldn't remember conversations. That was difficult for me. I used to lose words when I was about to speak them. I couldn't remember movies, so I got to watch them a second time! When I read a book, I could read it again because I didn't remember all the details. That was annoying. I knew my mind was slipping.

Things have improved in the last four years. I feel like my memory is getting better all the time. It is definitely not declining at any rate. I think I have stopped the downward spiral of cognitive impairment. As long as I don't get any worse, I can certainly live comfortably like I am right now. However, I know that my memory is continually improving. I am thinking clearly and I know my intelligence is acute. This week I was able to remember a phone number, the first time I've been able to remember a phone number since I can remember!

Some of Dr. Neal Barnard's recommendations for maintaining brain health are first and foremost, eat a whole food, no oil, plant-based diet.

You'll reduce your risk of Alzheimer's by 66%. Imagine that, reducing your risk, by that much, just by eating plants! You are changing your odds by just that one step alone. The next thing to do is to walk, 45 minutes, three times a week. I walk 45 minutes every day and I'm trying to get it up even higher. Eat berries, grapes, nuts and seeds every day. These are such simple things you can do to protect your brain, don't you think? And then, he suggests, you challenge your mind on a regular basis. Learn a language, do some puzzles - or even write a book!

Dr. Michael Greger, another one of my heroes, in his new book *How Not to Die*, says the spice saffron can help with memory loss. I've been looking for saffron in a tablet form. Dr. Greger suggests 500 mg per day. The latest scientific evidence suggests that saffron works better than one of the leading dementia drugs for returning your mind back to normal. Food is amazing, isn't it?

What I've learned from you, Judith, is that plant-based diets help to slow or reverse aging. That's because of the telomeres, the caps that are at the ends of the strands of DNA. As we age, as our cells age, those telomeres shorten. But what's been found is that when we switch to a whole food plant-based diet, over time the telomeres start to lengthen again.

Yes, Dr. Dean Ornish and other scientists have published some very interesting data on increasing telomere length with a plant-based diet along with other positive lifestyle changes. It's very encouraging research.

It's amazing! I know now I won't be getting Alzheimer's. Why is it that the general public still doesn't have this vital lifesaving information? My future is wide open with health and vitality because I am eating healthy now. I am so grateful to these doctor heroes: Dr. John McDougall, Dr. Neal Barnard, Dr. Caldwell Esselstyn, Dr. T. Colin Campbell, Dr. Dean Ornish, Dr. Michael Greger. They put their careers on the line and are fighting the establishment tooth and nail to get the truth out to the public, about the power of a whole food, plant-based diet to heal the body.

How has your life changed?

Oh, in every way. I have no pain. I don't take any medications or painkillers. I can move freely without joint restrictions. I can walk for miles and miles now. I have stamina and strength. I can do yoga. I have lost 53 pounds. I am not fat anymore, so I feel better about myself and of course I am healthier. I know I have stopped damaging my arteries. I know that all the sludge and plaque that built up in my arteries for 60 years is now clearing. The arteries to my brain are clearing. I know I will never have a heart attack or a stroke. I know I will never have to take blood pressure pills, cholesterol pills, diabetes pills, or painkillers for arthritis. I probably won't ever have to take any medical drugs for any condition because I won't be developing any more conditions! And, the icing on the cake is I know I never be getting Alzheimer's!

How are you feeling physically and mentally?

How do I feel? My happiness has gone through the roof. I am happy all the time. I feel relief. I feel hopeful. I am excited about the future. When you are living pain-free and have bountiful amounts of energy, and you lost all that weight, you feel wonderful. It is easy. Just eat potatoes, corn, rice, beans, fruits and vegetables, and your future is guaranteed to be healthy!

I'm going to get emotional here. I am extremely happy, because there was something that wasn't harmonious in my life. It is because of my love of animals. And I was eating them…..why didn't that….um…..why didn't I ever realize what I was doing? Why didn't I ever put two and two together? The lovely little Styrofoam package of meat that you buy at the grocery store was a living being, a couple of days ago, who probably suffered a horrible life and death in overcrowded conditions, confined in a dirty cage, never having stepped out in the sunlight. It never occurred to me.

The meat industry is a genius for being secretive about their affairs that go on behind closed doors. I'm not participating anymore. I am no longer supporting the inhumane treatment, the suffering and killing of animals. A hundred animals get to live this year and 100 more next year because I'm a vegan. That is 4000 animals by the end of my life that were not harmed on my behalf. For me, this is such a relief.

For 60 years of my life, it never occurred to me, I never connected the dots. Then all of a sudden, I'm not eating animals anymore and there is a peace in my soul. Eating my beautiful little friends was out of alignment with who I am. I feel like I'm living in harmony with my values now. By eating plants, I am living in complete non-violence, in peace with all Earth's creatures, with nature, with life. It is truly a remarkable feeling.

Also, I'm doing the most effective thing that has the most impact to stop hurting the earth. I am not contributing to factory farming. It is causing 51% of the world greenhouse gases. Did you know there are 150 billion animals slaughtered every year on our planet? This industry is what is causing these dangerous gases and global warming. This is what is polluting our water and using up all our natural resources of water, land, and forest. This is what is most likely going to wipe out all the life on our planet. You can stop the momentum of it by not eating meat anymore and not supporting factory farms. Simple, yet it's very effective.

Every single one of us can make a difference if we choose to. Each person can choose the food that heals their bodies. Those same foods that heal your body, heal the animals and heal the Earth with absolutely no extra effort. It all magically lines up. I just feel so much better. On every level, my quality of life is better, knowing that no animals have died for me to thrive. There's something so peaceful and beautiful about that.

What difficulties or obstacles have you faced?

Well, the biggest one I think is my family. I have a brother who I am very fond of, who lives in the Toronto area. He's got some growing health issues starting with arthritis in his neck and lower back. Another one is kidney stones. I am not allowed to talk with him about being a vegan because he loves his meat. People are emotionally attached to their food. This hurts me because I know he's going to die too young. I want to help him, but he can't hear me right now. He probably won't be able to hear me until he gets really sick. Two summers ago, we were up at his cottage, and I had to drive him three hours back to Toronto in the middle of the night because he was passing a kidney stone. He was in agony the whole way, and had to have it surgically removed. He gets sarcastic and defensive when I say anything about his food. That's been a challenge because I deeply care about him.

Also, the family that I live with, they all eat meat and dairy. To see the milk in the fridge, it drives me crazy! Young people think they are invincible, yet they are overweight, constipated, and developing health issues. They don't eat any fruits or vegetables. They eat bread and they eat meat. They won't listen to me. They think I'm just an eccentric old fool. I am looking forward to them moving out and getting their crap out of my fridge.

Now, interestingly enough, my 93-year-old father, watched me go from being a crippled girl with painful arthritis to being vibrant and disease-free. He witnessed my health improvement firsthand. He also watched his wife suffer, and he gets it. He's eating more the way I do. His health is great. He listens to me and I know I've influenced him.

There are three more challenges that I face. One of them is my doctor. I have a family doctor who is great for running blood tests, dispensing antibiotics, and giving the shingles vaccine, etc. She was indispensable when I was in a car accident many years ago, and I'm grateful for her care at that time. The problem is I can't find the kind of medical support I am really looking for, one who embraces this whole food, plant-based lifestyle. There are no vegan medical doctors in the city of Toronto, and the GTA (Greater Toronto Area), with a population of six million people! How could that be? I am on the hunt to find one. It's important to me.

I go to my doctor only to get my cholesterol, B_{12}, and thyroid levels checked. We absolutely do not see eye-to-eye on anything. She's all about pharmaceuticals, medical screening, and all that regular stuff. She has no idea that I stopped the progression of my arthritis with a plant-based diet, even though I have told her. So that's been really frustrating for me, because she doesn't value the information.

Another challenge is that I've been losing friends. I'm losing one right now. It's very hurtful. I am only guessing, but I think she is upset that I'm losing weight. She has been trying so hard for her entire adult life to lose weight and has had no success. Perhaps she is envious of my success. Perhaps she is sick of me talking about this awesome diet and that is why she is withdrawing from me. Six months ago, her knee was inflamed with arthritis and of course, I couldn't keep my mouth shut.

That is my field of expertise! She had made an appointment with her family doctor. A lot of good that is going to do! I said to her, "Why don't you try not eating meat and dairy for a week and see if it clears up?" She told me to shut up. She angrily said she would never stop eating meat until the day she dies. I said, "Well, then you are going to end up having a knee replacement like your father." That really annoyed her and she has been avoiding me ever since. I guess that didn't go well. Her daughter is vegan too. She is surrounded by the truth and isn't willing to change - well, not yet anyway!

The other thing is that our world is in trouble. As a whole community, a world community, we have to take action now because 50 years from now, environmental changes will be critical. I want to speak out. I haven't found my voice yet. I haven't found my stride. I talk about it when I'm out and about. I know people are turned off. I have to be quiet, or else I'm not going to have any friends left. I'm having difficulty trying to find my voice without upsetting people. I'm very frustrated about that. I just want to yell out at the world, "Wake up! Stop eating meat. By not supporting factory farms, it is the number one thing we can do to stop the greenhouse gases in our world." Being vegan is so unpopular and people don't want to hear it. They seem to be angry at you. Their face firms up as soon as you say you are vegan.

Where do you get your support from?

Initially, my support came from the internet. I love the stories on John McDougall's website. I go there for hours to read about his people. I listen to their videos there. I got my support from there, first of all, and then I finally decided I've got to find a group. I went to a Plant Pure Pod Meetup group. It's a vegan potluck meetup group that meets once a month here in Toronto. I've met some people there. That's where I found out about the Toronto Starch Solution meetup. When they said, there was a Starch Solution meetup in Toronto, I couldn't sleep, I was so excited. These are my people. You're doing the same as me. You are eating lots of starches and no oil! I was just so excited to meet you guys. I've only been to two meetings, but you are my people and I'm so glad to be here. Look what's happened, you and I are doing this project together. It's amazing.

How do you manage your food when you are at social events, weddings, parties, and barbecues?

I'm absolutely not good in restaurants. I would say I avoid eating out because when I go out, I think, "Well, it's going to be a cheese night." It seems that all you can get that does not have meat, is cheese pasta. That's pretty well it. I'm not the kind of personality that will demand the chef create something special for me. I don't like to ruffle people's feathers. Instead I'll have a little cheese, which I'm working on not doing. So, it's avoidance, that's how I do it. (Update: since this interview, Diane has learned to ask for dairy-free food in restaurants.)

I always carry food in the car. Always. I won't be stuck when lunch rolls around without something to eat. When I go to people's houses I bring my own food. I just bring my own little portion.

I eat really simple. I'm not the greatest cook. I'm not really interested in cooking. I like to get it over with. It is a chore to me. Let's get it done, so I can get on to what I really want to do. So, I eat really simple and I really enjoy my food. As John McDougall says, you can put a little salt and pepper on your potatoes. To me, that makes it delicious. That's all I need. I have my pile of potatoes with a bit of salt and pepper. Sometimes, I'll cut up a little dill, and sometimes I'll put a little bit of onion on top, and it's just over the moon delicious for me. I have my steamed vegetables. I have my rice maker, and I throw my steamed vegetables in there. They're done in ten minutes. I have my steamed spinach every night which I just love, and that's it. I make it simple.

One thing that really helped me was Mary McDougall's Mini. Mary is Dr. McDougall's wife. She has a YouTube video, where she talks about eating just one starch, like potatoes, and nothing else for a week. Just try it, and then you'll see how you can make your life simple. That was an "aha" moment for me. I tried it. I only lasted a couple of days though and then I wanted to have my vegetables and my fruit as well. It taught me that you can eat so simply, like unbelievably simple. You can have porridge four times a day. If you're hungry at midnight, you can have a pile of potatoes and you're not breaking any rules. You can eat when you're hungry, and you can stuff yourself with starch. You can be satisfied and you never have to go hungry again. That's what that taught me, that little exercise of hers, Mary McDougall's Mini. You don't have to be a gourmet chef to do this. Eat potatoes three times a day. I eat porridge at least two times a day because I love it and it satisfies my hunger. Simple things work best, like a pile of rice, you know. I put a little salt on that, and it makes it so yummy.

What advice do you have for beginners?

I love what Dr. Neal Barnard recommends to beginners in his Quick Start Program. You start off by taking a week and observing all the things that are plant-based that you like such as pancakes, porridge, fruits and nuts on your cereal, and almond milk. You look at all the things you could eat for dinner like pasta with marinara sauce, bean tacos, etc. You gather up ideas for a number of dishes and foods that you know you're going to eat for breakfast, lunch, and dinner. Then, in the second week, you dive in. You go in one hundred percent. By going all in, for three weeks, you're going to see a big difference in how you feel. You have to go all in, no cheating. You are going to feel the results of this way of eating. Your ailments are going to start improving. You are going to have energy like you wouldn't believe, and you are probably going to lose some weight. With my arthritis, if I didn't go all in, I never would have seen any of the results that I got.

Secondly, my advice to those who are just starting, if you do goof up, be kind to yourself but get right back on the program. Don't waste your energy being upset with yourself. Just get back on the program, the very next time you eat.

Some other advice is to get all the junk food, meats and dairy out of the house, so they are not there tempting you in weak moments. My family has their junk food, like pie, cookies and pastries piled right on the counter. It's right there in the kitchen on the counter. I walk by it a hundred times a day, and at one point I just put a note to myself on the cookie package. "This is not healthy. Your joints will seize!" Now I'm past that. That garbage can stay there on the counter and it doesn't tempt me anymore. It would have been so much easier if it wasn't there at all. I still crave chocolate once in awhile, and if I indulge, I'll pay the next day with inflammation. You do the best you can to follow the plan. There will be weak moments. Forgive yourself and climb right back on.

What are your future goals?

When my Dad does his transition, I will have to move out of this house. My intention is to buy a little farm property. I don't know where yet. I'm kind of taken with BC (British Columbia), but my kids are here in Toronto, so it will probably be somewhere close by.

I love to garden, and I've never grown my own organic vegetables. That would be one thing I want to experience. I tried to sneak some corn and other veggies in the backyard garden this year but the squirrels fought me for it, and they won! With a farm, my intention is to have a big organic garden that I can live off. That's what I want to try, even if I only do it for a year or two. I just want to experience that.

I'd also like to rescue a few farm animals. I figure I owe them that much. I've never had an herbivore pet. That covers a lot of pets. That could be a goat, a sheep, a pig, a cow, a horse, a camel, an alpaca, and a rabbit. I want to rescue a few. Living out in the country, it would really be nice to have a couple of horses. I think I'd like to take in a couple of race horses. Like the greyhound dogs, the race horses are discarded when they're done racing. You can get them for nothing. It would be nice just to give them a home for the rest of their lives. I'd take in a lame horse or a blind one. I don't want to ride them or anything, just give them a home.

Yes, instead of them being euthanized at the age of six, because they're injured and they can't race anymore.

It's the saddest thing what they do to horses. Oh my God, it's tragic. What they do to greyhound dogs as well is awful. But, we won't go there today. I intend on rescuing a few animals. Not too many, just a few. I want to see what their personalities are like. It's going to be a whole new adventure. That's a future dream of mine, to have a little farm.

How do you see yourself changing the world?

Well, I am co-writing this book. Perhaps we will start another vegan meetup group in the west end of Toronto. It's about speaking up. By not being quiet anymore, we're going to spread the word.

Also, I have a friend, who is a computer wizard, and she wants to do t-shirts and designs on mugs and sell them on the internet. I am very excited about doing a series of vegan designs, about health, animal rights, and saving the planet.

I have some plans for my children and they don't know it yet. They both have health issues. My kids are 29 and 27 years old. They both have irritable bowel syndrome. I would love to get them down to McDougall's program for ten days. I bet that the IBS would clear up in those ten days. Health is so important. According to them, I am an active member of a vegan cult. They snicker at me, but they have no idea that I'm much more evolved I am than they are! Young people think they know everything. When I have my little farm, they're going to be out there getting fresh vegetables from my garden and finding out those lovely little animals have personalities, like those baby goats and lambs that are rescued.

I took my kids to the Wishing Well Animal Sanctuary last fall. A couple of weeks earlier, I went there with a few friends. We had a wonderful time interacting with the animals. Everybody who works here is a vegan. It is a beautiful small farm. They have about 150 rescued animals with very sad stories. There is a little herd of sheep, some goats, and a lot of pigs. They have a whole herd of cattle, three horses and a llama.

I was telling my son how excited I was about this place, and how I had never touched a cow in my life. I ate a lot of cows but I'd never touched one or looked her in the eye or offered her something to eat. There was this one friendly cow, a jersey cow, and she likes people. She was visiting with everybody.

There are lots of wonderful things coming for me in my life. There's growing vegetables and rescuing a few animals. There's saving my children, and saving the planet through designing t-shirts, and through leadership at groups and meetups. We are speaking up through this book project. We're forming this community, and this community is going to grow throughout the world. We're going to convert some people. We're going to find our voices and we're going to speak out, loud and clear, and we're going to back it with the latest science.

Chapter Seven
Lori

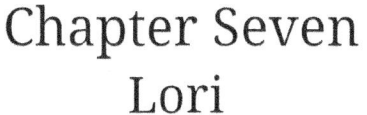

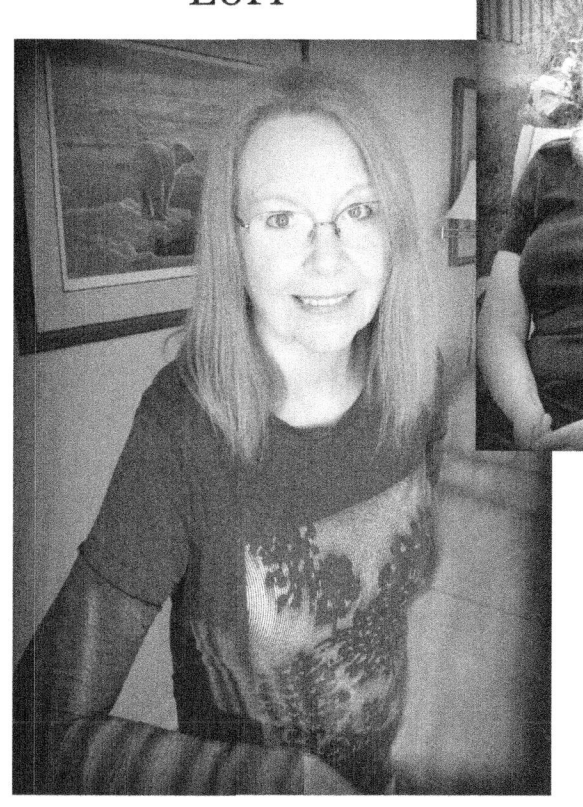

Lori was stressed and exhausted, dragging herself to and from her difficult job, when her doctor discovered her diabetes. Other health problems were starting to rear their ugly heads too, like high blood pressure, sciatica, and fibromyalgia. Then the unthinkable happened. Lori had three stokes. Lori has been following the McDougall plan faithfully for just over a year now and has reversed most of her chronic conditions and lost over 35 pounds.

Toronto Starch Solution Meetup Group
Group Toronto Starch Solution Meetup

Chapter Seven - Lori's Interview

Can you tell us a bit about your background, your work, your family and your interests?

My interests always have been nutrition. Since I was 17, I was going to a health food store and buying organic stuff, way back in the seventies and people thought I was nuts. Then the eighties came along, and like everybody, I lost sight of nutrition. I was drinking and partying, and of course, I was getting confused by the information we were getting like on olive oil and Caesar salads. I didn't have to watch my diet at all, because I was very healthy.

Then, my thirties came along. My daughter was born when I was 32 years old, and I got really, really sick with toxemia. It almost killed me. It almost killed both of us. I was in the hospital for 17 days, on complete bed rest, but it didn't control the blood pressure. I had to have an emergency C-section. Of course, now, looking back on it, I realize it was all diet-related. I am sure of it. Of course, the doctors wouldn't tell you that.

After the birth of my daughter, I completely recovered, and my blood pressure went back to normal. I was healthy in my forties. I didn't go to the doctor for many years. I remember my fasting blood sugar was totally normal and my blood pressure was normal. I was busy with what I was doing at the time. I had morphed from executive assistant and got my real estate licence and was trying to do real estate full-time. I was under a tremendous amount of stress with the real estate career.

Looking back on it, I thought, it wasn't stress, it was diabetes and I didn't know it. Now, I know it by the symptoms I was having.

By the time I did go to the doctor, I was around 50 years old. I had blood tests done. I was busy, busy, busy. I got a call from the doctor's office. The receptionist said, "The doctor wants to see you." I'm thinking, "But I just saw her." I said, "I'm busy. I am working on some deals." She goes, "No, the doctor wants to see you." I thought, it's cancer or something. I went to see her and she was very grave in her demeanour and she told me that I was sick. She said, "Your blood sugars are off the chart, your triglycerides are three times higher than they're supposed to be. You have diabetes." I guess I had probably been diabetic for about a year before I even got diagnosed. I decided not to take the medication recommended to me. I said, "Give me three months and I'll beat this."

I went to the Naturopathic College and found a naturopath. The naturopath put me on a plan which strangely enough included olive oil and fish. I also had to take supplements that you wouldn't believe, and that I had never heard of. But you know, it worked, even with the olive oil and the fish. I went back to see the doctor. I went back about four months later. She said, "If I didn't know you were diabetic, I wouldn't even think these were your blood results." She asked, "What are you doing?" I said "I am taking olive oil right off the spoon. I am taking lecithin granules, I am taking these supplements and those supplements, and eating salmon three times a week, right out of a can." Apparently canned salmon was good. She said, "Well you can't keep this up." I said, "Oh yeah, sure I can." She said, "No, I don't think it is sustainable." And, she was right.

I slipped off the wagon and my results got worse. I was resisting taking the oral medications for diabetes and then I finally broke down and started taking them. I took them for a short period of time, because they cause extreme gastrointestinal problems. I don't know if you have talked to anybody who takes Metformin, but you can't even leave the house, you have such diarrhea. I just stopped taking it. I went back to see her and I thought, I am not taking this. I need a life. That is when we decided to put me on insulin. My body and my instincts told me, I'd rather take insulin than take oral medications. I guess that is one of the reasons why I love Dr. McDougall so much, because he concurs totally. He says he takes everybody off the oral medications because they have such extreme side effects. I have been on insulin for about five years now. Murray, my ex-husband and I, have tried everything. We are both diabetic and we both have high blood pressure. We both have high cholesterol. By the way Murray is my ex-husband but we are best friends and we live in the same house.

We tried the Paleo diet. We just made so many detours in our health before we found Dr. McDougall. All the literature, all the articles, and all the books say that if you are diabetic, you should be eating a low carbohydrate diet. This seemed to make sense. We were eating lots and lots of vegetables and lots of meat. Yes, your blood does get better for a while, but eventually, things go south.

Because you are eating a lot more vegetables with a low carb diet, it is better, but it is not the ideal way of eating. It is an improvement. Then, your blood starts to go up again and as soon as you throw any carbs into the mix your blood sugar goes off the charts. I said to Murray, "Well I guess you can never cheat and have some rice or potatoes or anything." What I know now, is we have clogged up all our cells with fat, and the insulin can't get into the cells. Anytime we ate any carbs it was insane.

How did I find McDougall? I really don't know. It must have been fate. I saw the movie, *Forks over Knives*. Isn't that how it always starts? I have Netflix and I was looking for something to watch. I like documentaries and this movie struck me as something that looks interesting. I'll watch it because it had to do with diet and the environment. That's what started it all. From this movie, I started looking for other people's videos on YouTube. I found Dr. Neal Barnard first. I didn't find Dr. McDougall right away. Neal Barnard looks at the causes of diabetes and I looked at the title, *Program for Reversing Diabetes*, and it jumped out at me. He was talking about the cause of diabetes being the fat in the cells. Then, Dr. Caldwell Esselstyn, I watched his videos about the damage eating oil causes to your arteries and cells. He is quite humorous in his delivery and he was featured in the movie, *Forks over Knives*. Then, there was Dr. T. Colin Campbell. I watched some of his things. I have such respect for that man. He almost lost his career for just telling the truth.

I followed a link to Dr. McDougall's website. It had something directly to do with diabetes. I went down the right-hand side where he has all the success stories. I watched all the videos of people who had reversed their diabetes. There was one story of success after another. As I was watching these things, I was thinking, "Hey I think there is something to this." I am willing to try it. We have tried everything else. Murray and I have tried the Paleo diet, Weight Watchers, and the Bernstein diet. Murray, in fact, had tried everything.

I remember buying the book, *The Starch Solution* by Dr. John McDougall, and I know for a fact it was in February of 2016 because I found the receipt tucked into the book. We had stopped eating meat already because we were following the *Forks over Knives Plan*. I had bought the two books, *Forks over Knives Plan* and *Forks over Knives - The Cook Book*. We were basically following a low-fat vegan diet, which is similar to Dr. McDougall's diet. It was slightly different and we were having some success and already losing weight by February.

I bought the book, *The Starch Solution* and we started following it and have never looked back. We bought Dr. Joel Fuhrman's book *Eat to Live*, too. I don't know how many books I bought. I bought them all. Somebody has got to have the answer here!

We had made quite a few of the recipes out of *Forks over Knives - The Cook Book*. We tried Dr. Fuhrman's recipes. We loved Dr. Fuhrman's Caesar salad dressing. We were making some of Dr. McDougall's recipes. I said to Murray, "Which one of these people or philosophies do you feel is the best?" Murray has a gift of being able to sort through things, taking the nuggets, and simplifying it. He said, "You know, out of all them, the simplest and easiest to follow is Dr. McDougall. He just makes it simple. You don't have to spend the afternoon in the kitchen."

Like some of the *Forks over Knives* recipes, while they might be delicious, they are complicated, and you spend a lot of time pureeing, grinding, and blending stuff together. Murray said, "I would never do this by myself. If you weren't here and we weren't cooking together, it would be far too complicated. I like Dr. McDougall's philosophy. Keep it simple. Brown rice, potatoes, steamed veggies, and you're okay."

There is this thing in my head about getting enough nutrients. I am always worried I am not going to get enough and I'm not going to be okay. This can't possibly be a balanced diet, eating only potatoes, beans, rice, porridge, fruits, and vegetables. I must be missing something. It has taken me months to get it into my head that this is a very healthy way to eat that is nutrient dense. It is a lifetime of conditioning and worrying that I must be missing something. No, you are going to be fine, that is all the human body needs. I finally understand this now, but it took me a long time to really get it. All of a sudden, something relaxed inside of me and now I get it, that this is all you need.

And, more than that, this diet is optimal! You couldn't eat any better if you tried.

Yet the message that we get is all confusing and conflicting. This week, you can eat eggs, next week, you can't eat eggs. Now, you can eat eggs again. Peanut butter is good for you. Peanut butter is bad for you. Meat is good for you, meat is bad for you. It is just so confusing. And then, I would get the *Vitality Magazine* and the *Alive Magazine* and again, I don't know where they are getting their information from, but now I am sceptical. Before, they used to be my bible with the latest studies showing bla bla bla. I have been following nutrition my whole life, and yet, I am thoroughly confused. It makes me angry because it affected me personally. I was very sick when I was pregnant, not to mention the last 10-11 years of my life with diabetes and the effect that this misinformation has had on me.

I have had three strokes directly related to the diabetes, and I am feeling frustrated and angry. It upsets me to think that this misinformation was naively put out there without being regulated or released responsibly. I think there are vested interests that purposefully put that information out there, just to confuse people, for their own gain, just to make a profit. I can see why Dr. McDougall is so frustrated too. I just watched a video on YouTube this morning, the one that Dr. McDougall calls *Child Abuse*. We are making our kids sick with malnutrition and eating the wrong foods. As a grandmother, I am concerned, because my grandson is sick like my daughter was sick as a baby.

I was desperate to help her when she was a baby. I took her off cow's milk. I investigated a lot of alternative stuff because she was throwing up constantly. It was a Chinese Canadian doctor who finally said to me, she is probably allergic to cow's milk. None of the other doctors had told me that. She threw up constantly until she was almost two so he said, "You might try goat's milk." This was back in the 1980s. We were living in Keswick. I had to drive all the way to Newmarket to a health food store to get the goat's milk. That solved my daughter's problem. Once she got to a certain age, where she didn't need a bottle anymore, I switched her to soy milk.

That was a blessing getting her off cow's milk so young.

My daughter had put my grandson on cow's milk. He was having terrible, terrible ear infections. I can understand the disconnect with my daughter, because she doesn't remember how sick she was with cow's milk. She used to have terrible ear infections too. Anyway, he is on soy milk now, but it took her a long time to do it. You know, none of those infections would ever have happened if she had put him on soy milk in the first place.

Don't you think it is really hard to be a parent because of all the peer pressure and the brainwashing by big business and their advertising?

You are so afraid that you are doing some damage to your child by going against the grain. The worst thing a mother wants to do is injure her child. My child might be deficient in something.

I remember going to a doctor when my daughter was very young. I told the doctor I had taken her off cow's milk and put her on soy milk. I got the distinct feeling the doctor wanted to charge me with child abuse because this woman isn't giving her child the socially acceptable cow's milk. She was saying to me, "You need to put her back on it." I was saying, "You don't understand what we went through, ear infections, trips to the hospital, constantly throwing up. Her stomach was all bloated like a little kid from Biafra. That all went away when she stopped drinking cow's milk. I am not putting her back on it." There's a doctor for you.

Imagine the kind of tenacity you had to have at the time, to seek alternatives for your suffering child and go against the establishment. That is very impressive, Lori. I hope you know that now.

After that, I learned not to tell doctors too much, not to share too much. That was a weird, weird session. I think she was going to fill out paperwork and have somebody come to my house. I was scared. I was frightened because she was very hostile to me. She didn't quite put it into words, about "damaging your child", but she was almost accusing me of some form of abuse. I have never forgotten that.

What improvements in your health and weight have you had so far?

I asked Murray this question because he is the one that sees me. He said, "You are thinking clearer. Your mind is sharper. You are more fit. You have more energy. You have a greater sense of well-being." I feel so good. My energy is off the charts! I just love my potatoes and Mary McDougall's gravy, and some brown rice, and I feel so satisfied and satiated. That is the thing with *The Starch Solution*, you are not hungry all the time, opening the fridge up and looking for something to eat.

It is wonderful being a McDougaller! I attended another vegan potluck. I remember somebody brought a salad and it was smothered in oil. After being committed to eating the McDougall way, I am finding the oil in food disgusting. You find that feeling of it in your mouth, it is awful now.

I was getting desperate to meet other vegan people. I felt so isolated and misunderstood. I was willing to meet any vegetarian. I was in seventh heaven when I found *The Starch Solution* meetup in Toronto! Imagine, there are other people who eat the same as me in this city!

There were the five of us McDougallers at this non-McDougall vegan event. There was that woman who said, "Oh, I never eat carbs." She said, "It just turns to sugar in your bloodstream." I thought, I would have probably said the same thing five years ago.

Did your numbers improve? Tell us about that.

I used to take 30 units of insulin, now I only take 10. I have been able to reduce these amounts by two thirds. I think I am, according to Dr. McDougall, type 1.5 diabetic. I don't want to be pessimistic, but I think, after all these months, I would have hoped to be off all the insulin. Maybe after the age of 60, your body doesn't have the ability to recover like it used to. But hey, I am fine with this.

But you're not done yet. You don't know what's coming.

Yeah, I don't know. Murray and I just went on the really strict plan, *The McDougall Program for Maximum Weight Loss*. I just bought that book three weeks ago and marked passages for Murray to do his homework, so he reads and understands the concepts. You know, we have been following *The Starch Solution* plan, which would be fine for someone who is not diabetic. There are still a lot of tofu recipes in there and we both love tofu, but it is 45% fat. We were eating it like crazy. We were still eating too much fat. We both have noticed a big improvement since we have been on the stricter version of *The Starch Solution*. You are right, I am not finished yet. Give me another few months and see if I can get off the rest of this insulin.

We were starting to get discouraged with *The Starch Solution* because our weight loss had reached a plateau, and we still had lots of weight to lose. It was hard not to feel disappointed. We had watched all the success videos and we were following the program perfectly, but we couldn't say that our numbers were improving as much as we hoped. In retrospect, I think we can use *The Starch Solution* program as the maintenance diet once we reach our medical and physical targets and get cured. Until we get our optimal weight and health back, we have to do the McDougall Program for Maximum Weight Loss.

Murray was surprised when I came home with yet another book. "You bought another book?" I said "Yes!" He said, "How many books are you going to buy?" I said, "I was sitting at the Indigo book store and I was reading it, and there was too much information to absorb so I bought it because I can't remember all this information we need." I said, "It was worth it because there is a lot of information in that book that is different from *The Starch Solution*."

For a person with chronic health issues, this book, *The McDougall Program for Maximum Weight Loss* is important. The tofu recipes which I was really happy with were not supporting our recovery from diabetes because of the fat content. I love tofu and we shouldn't have been eating it. I don't remember reading that in *The Starch Solution* but Dr. McDougall talks about it directly in the McDougall Program for Maximum Weight Loss book. We were sitting there eating big slabs of tofu. No wonder we were not losing any weight. Who knew? I am not blaming him. I am just saying, I am glad we discovered it.

I lost 20 pounds with *The Starch Solution* and then the weight loss levelled off. I said I have got to get rid of the rest of this. I am tired of being a fat vegan after two years of being on *The Starch Solution* program. I got the book, *The McDougall Program for Maximum Weight Loss* and I lost 16 more pounds.

There is quite a difference between the books. You take out flour, nuts, seeds, and tofu. I went extreme and took out my ground flax seed that I sprinkle on my cereal every morning. We were doing Dr. Fuhrman's Caesar salad dressing, which we love. We had to cut that out too. We both used to love Caesar salad made with olive oil and egg. The base of Fuhrman's Caesar dressing was cashews and sesame seeds, and then you use almond milk. It is so delicious with lots of garlic and I was using kelp to give it that anchovy flavour, but I told Murray we can't even have that anymore. Those cashews, man, who knew? We were allowed a handful of nuts in *The Starch Solution*, but now, we don't eat any nuts.

Murray had to give up his bread, his beloved bread. He is a habitual person. He takes his sandwich every day to work. I don't have a problem with giving that up. He was eating Yves fake meat and it was a huge transition for him to give up his daily sandwich. I said, "No more sandwiches." I was very proud of him after he got over the shock. He was very, very reluctant to give them up, so it is just temporary, while we follow this program. He is taking potatoes, brown rice, beans, and a salad to work. He feels like he can do that. If he had refused to give up the bread, there wouldn't be any more weight loss. He had hit this plateau for about a month or so, and he had stopped losing weight. The weight loss is what keeps you going.

You look and feel fantastic! Also, your skin looks good.

My grandmother used to use the expression, "You are sickening for something." You can tell by somebody's colour if they are off. People just look at you, after you have been eating this way, and see that you are more vibrant, have vitality and health.

What is your total weight loss?

Fed Up with Being Fat and Sick

I lost 35 pounds. I was pretty heavy. I was 160 last year, and today, I am 126. I may have to start adding a little bit of tofu and nuts back into my diet so I don't lose any more, but I am still going to continue with *The McDougall Program for Maximum Weight Loss* to support Murray. I will do this with him until he reaches his goal weight. I also want to get all the fat out of my cells to cure my diabetes, and I think I still have some. I must completely clean the fat out of my cells.

What kind of foods do you eat daily?

Potatoes! I eat plenty of potatoes, brown rice, Mary McDougall's gravy, berries, oatmeal, and not too many fruits. Murray got me on oatmeal. He eats it religiously every morning. I didn't want to eat oatmeal. I'd rather eat toast but now that I am not eating bread anymore, I joined Murray in eating porridge. It's good.

I'm stuck on my Instant Pot. You've got to get one! It's a life changer. Murray's oatmeal would be sputtering all over the stove and he'd be cooking it for 45 minutes because he likes the steal cut oats. With the Instant Pot, you put it in and it cooks in just three minutes. You wait another 10 minutes to let the pressure go down. That's it, you're done! It's so creamy and delicious. If there is anything you are going to do for yourself this year, treat yourself to an Instant Pot.

We have been buying a lot of canned beans and beans aren't cheap any more, four dollars for a can of organic beans now. Remember when beans were dirt cheap? As soon as we use up all our cans in the pantry, I am going to make all our own beans in the Instant Pot and then freeze them. For brown rice, it turns out perfectly too. I make brown rice, enough for four days at once, so you are cutting down your cooking time in the kitchen to practically nothing. It turns out so beautifully. I am doing rice, beans and potatoes in the Instant Pot. Oh my God, the potatoes are just so perfect, soft, and beautiful.

The first time I used the Instant Pot, I made Chef AJ's red lentil chili and the workmen were here installing the new doors. The one workman said, "Oh my God, you are killing me here with whatever you are cooking. It smells fantastic. I love garlic." When it was done, I asked him if he wanted some and he said, "Yes. I didn't think you would ever ask." I served him a bowl of chili. "Oh my God, this is fantastic." I told him we are vegan and he said, "I don't believe in veganism, but I have to tell ya, this is the best vegan chili I have ever had." That was a fun experience to remember.

What have been the some of the challenges? What foods have you had a hard time giving up?

I had a hard time giving up cheese of course. I hear that a lot from women. I could give up meat really easily, but real cheddar cheese in a sandwich with tomato and mayo was hard to give up. Yeah, cheese, but now I am okay. The craving is gone. Once in awhile, we go to a restaurant and have a vegan pizza with Daiya cheese and I'm good with that, because it's just occasionally. I could give up eggs easily. I could give up the meat. It was the cheese. Dr. Neal Barnard says there are opiates in the cheese. It seems like everybody is suffering with the cheese. Ask any vegan. That's what it is. I am over that now. It took me a while and I don't even think about it anymore.

I haven't had it in so long I wonder what would happen if I did have a real piece as opposed to the Daiya. I have to tell you, Murray and I went and had our first pizza in town, here at the Pizzaiolo. We had the pizza with the Daiya cheese, and we wolfed that pizza down, it was so good. He said, "As long as I can get this once in a while, I can do this vegan thing. I won't miss cheese." Daiya has got that formula down pat. I am sure it's not low-fat, but man, it tastes great and it's not laced with animal products. If we only do it once in awhile, why not? This is my treat.

Are there any challenges with family and friends?

No, I have been to some family dinners and they noticed the weight loss, and were concerned initially because I hadn't seen my brothers and sisters for awhile. I think they were wondering what the hell I was doing. Since then, they have heard Murray's story. He was at the last family thing. I told them that he is off all these medications, and at this point, he has lost about 80 pounds. He has lost 13 more since then. When they saw him, it was a wow. Are they going to do it? Nope. I don't expect them to.

I would say the biggest challenge is when I go to my meetup groups. When I go to the pub to go dancing, I made the mistake of mentioning it to a couple of people, and of course, I get the lecture. "Well, people are meant to be meat eaters. That is how we developed as a species and developed our brains, our big carnivore brains. Or, where do you get your fat from?" I said, "I am still eating almonds and sesame seeds and chia seeds." They nod, and then the ubiquitous question they ask next is, "Where do you get your protein from?" and, "What about calcium?" I am so glad somebody asked. Or "Where do you get your iron?" I said, "At my age I don't need iron." And they said, "Oh, everybody needs iron." I said, "I am eating beans and legumes and tofu. Spinach is a good source of iron." Oh yes, I am just so glad somebody asked me that question. Everybody wants to know, where do you get your protein?

There is a t-shirt out there that says, "Don't ask me about my protein and I won't ask you about your cholesterol."

I want that one! If I ever see that, I am going to get it. We got the Dr. Greger one that says, "Plant Powered". I live in the city. I don't want to get into a fight with somebody on the subway because they don't like what my t-shirt says.

You are retired, at the moment, so you don't have any co-workers giving you a hard time, and you are so lucky you and your husband are doing this together.

Yes. I thank God. He has been my validation, my supporter, and it just gives me such a sense of satisfaction that I have been able to help him. I said thank God this is working for him, because he was kind of my experiment. If it hadn't worked, that would have been bad. We are seeing such amazing results. For all his life, he has struggled with his weight and health, and we didn't understand what we were doing wrong. We'd be eating a meal with a piece of meat, some vegetables, and a small bit of potatoes, and couldn't lose the weight and were starving. Who knew? We were always hungry and always depriving ourselves for years and years. The worst part was beating yourself up for being unsuccessful, like you did something wrong, and accusing yourself of not having enough will power.

I have never experienced what Murray experienced, which is being morbidly obese. Imagine the frustration of not knowing what you are doing wrong. He tried so many different diets like Dr. Bernstein's. All these different things that he tried and none of them worked. Finally, we found McDougall's program and it actually works.

The other day, Murray was still sitting here and I could tell he was still hungry. We had had brown rice, spinach, and cauliflower. He didn't want any more, but I knew he was still hungry. I could tell. It is just second nature to deny himself. I went into the house and got him some more. He had another bowl of rice with some gravy on it and then he said, "I am so full." I didn't want him to be ravenous at 11 p.m. because he didn't eat enough at 6 p.m.

Dr. Doug Lisle explains it so perfectly. I have learned so much from those YouTube videos. To be ravenous at midnight means you haven't eaten enough during the day. I have experienced that too being on *The Starch Solution*. I thought I had eaten enough, but at around 10 p.m., I am hungry again and I start searching for something to eat. As a diabetic, it is bad to eat at bedtime. It's because you haven't eaten enough during the day. I get that. I can relate to this.

I often have a bowl of steal cut oats with berries at bedtime.

That's what I had last night with no berries. It takes away the hunger, and it is good for us.

How would you say Dr. McDougall has changed your life?

Oh my God, I feel like a different person now. I have so much more energy. I discovered quite by accident, while I was being diagnosed with the stroke symptoms, that I have fibromyalgia. I said, "No I don't. My sister has it. I don't. I have enough problems with diabetes." The doctor said, "No you really do have it because every trigger point that I have pushed, you are sore." There were days when my whole body ached, but I figured that was just fatigue or diabetes or whatever. Since I changed to Dr. McDougall's plan, it is nonexistent. I have upped my carbs to 80 percent of my diet. We try to do 80-10-10. I think your muscles are starving for glycogen. I can remember dragging myself through supermarkets to buy groceries and realized my whole body was aching. I thought it was an old age thing. I don't have that anymore.

How has this changed my life? I have ridiculous, just ridiculous amounts of energy. My stamina is better. I have better digestion. I am sleeping better. I feel more optimistic. I have a sense of hope that I didn't have before. I have a sense of hope that I can actually reverse this diabetes. At the minimum, at least maintain this level of just ten units of insulin and not have it progress. This McDougall lifestyle plan is easy to maintain. I have never had this before, a diet that is satisfying me and promoting my health.

Hope is a big deal. You are not going to have to go through the horrible end stages of diabetes that slowly kills you.

Like losing a toe, and then losing your eyesight next. It is a sense of hope and a sense of achievement. Just by changing my diet, I have accomplished this, and a sense of purpose that I can help other people like I have helped my husband. Everywhere I go, when I get a chance, I talk about Dr. McDougall and try to get people onto his website.

I went to a restaurant on Danforth Avenue. It was a pizza place and I told the waitress I don't want any oil with the salad dressing. I said that I am vegan and she said that I can't have the salad dressing because there is honey in the salad dressing. I thanked her for correcting me. I shouldn't say vegan. I am plant-based. She wanted to know what was left to eat? I told her everything, potatoes, sweet potatoes. I rhymed off a list of things I can eat. She thought that was interesting. I brought up Dr. McDougall because I always do and she said her girlfriend just got diagnosed with MS. Her doctor put her on a low-fat diet. I told her to read Dr. McDougall's article on a low-fat diet and MS. He has been telling people for 25 years that a low-fat diet is highly recommended for people with MS. I am glad to hear that the doctors have actually told her to go on a low-fat diet. She wrote drcdougall.com down. I told her to make sure her girlfriend looks at this. She might be able to tweak her diet even more and cure her condition.

Who knows what her doctors consider low-fat. It probably isn't the same as what you and I would consider low-fat. She might still be drinking skim milk. She might still be eating eggs but just the egg whites and take the yolks out. I don't know what her doctor is telling her. At least, they have come that far to say low-fat. MS is such a debilitating disease. It is another horrible one, and she has three small kids. If it is in the early stages, it could be completely reversed with McDougall's diet. I hope she gives the information to her friend.

I had Dr. McDougall's book back in the nineties. Murray was struggling with his weight and I got one of McDougall's books, and we tried a few recipes. Both of us were going out for breakfast and having bacon and eggs, and French toast, and all that stuff. I remember selling the book at a garage sale. Who knew? He was trying to come through. You know what I mean? The knowledge tries to come to you but it's whether you grab it or not.

Do you have any advice for beginners?

Yeah, keep it simple. What I learned is that it's okay and healthy to just keep it simple. You are okay with some potatoes and a vegetable or a bit of brown rice or porridge in the morning. You are okay.

Secondly, for beginners, travel with your own food. When you travel, carry your own salad dressing. I find salads are the hardest thing. You are out in a restaurant and you tell the waitress you want fat-free dressing. I don't even want the fat-free dressing that is out there. It is full of chemicals and stuff.

What do you do when you go to parties?

Eat before you go out and then you won't worry about what is there. I haven't done a lot of socializing except the pub nights. All they have is calamari and chicken wings where I go. I can't have any of it so I eat before I go.

Be careful who you talk to about this new way of eating. I had a guy get hostile with me about it. And so the story goes, it is because we ate meat that our brains developed. Yeah, but yours didn't develop too far.

Where did they come up with that anyway? Some scientist said that at the Smithsonian Institute. Yet evidence is showing through DNA that we were herbivores for the longest time. Dr. Barnard says in one of his videos that humans are actually really bad hunters. The average person could not catch an animal. Then, we got smarter and set snares up but in the early days it was rare to eat an animal. I can't imagine running after an animal and catching it and killing it. We are just not designed for that.

If you were going to a dinner party, a wedding, or a social event, how would you handle that?

Eat before. At a wedding, I'd be very selective about what I would choose from the buffet. Fill up as much as I could on the low-fat stuff. I'd tough it out until I could leave, and then go to my car where I'd have something good to eat.

I went to a funeral and when it was all done, I went to the car and had something to eat. There were two other vegans there too. I heard one of the gals say, "I'm hungry. I'm going to go get our food out of the car."

I think that is a really good tip for beginners because we didn't know that in the beginning. Always travel with your own food. Don't stress that you are getting enough nutrients because you are. It is actually the ideal diet.

I heard Dr. McDougall say if you are eating potatoes that is all you need. The potato has everything you need nutritionally. If you are eating rice, you have to add a piece of broccoli.

There's this fellow named Andrew Taylor from Australia, and he is a school teacher. He made the decision to eat only potatoes for one whole year. You can find him on YouTube under the name Spud Fit. Nobody will be able to dispute that potatoes aren't healthy ever again. A doctor is tracking his numbers as he goes along, to make sure he is operating at an optimal level. He is proving conclusively that you can live off potatoes. Whether they choose to believe it and incorporate it, that's their business, but at least they can't disprove it. He is doing a great service. You could see it gave Dr. McDougall hope.

I hope Dr. McDougall lives to see his work validated and be accepted by the medical community in the next ten years or so. He has tried so hard for so many years. Maybe he feels like he has failed, but he really hasn't. He has been instrumental in getting the word out about the truth of a plant-based diet to the Western world.

How has your daughter reacted to her parents doing this?

She hasn't seen Murray in person since last summer, but the last time we Skyped, she said "Dad how much are you down to now? I can tell the difference in your face." Since then, he is deliberately staying behind the camera because he wants to surprise her when he sees her at the end of this month. When she sees him, she is going to be amazed. She is on board with it. She sees the improvement in both of us. The evidence is clear. We are both hoping she will follow us because she is struggling with her weight since she had her two children. She has about 40 or so pounds to lose. We bought her a copy of *The Starch Solution*, and we are taking it out to her.

We have told a lot of people. Everybody asks Murray what he is doing. This is amazing. He has lost 110 pounds. But are they going to do it? Probably not. The catalyst for us was our emergency health situation.

What about you doctor? Is he on board?

He is a new doctor. He is a young male of Indian background. I figure he has lots of vegetarian relatives. I am sure he probably does. When I saw him my average blood sugar had gone from 8.4 to 7. He wanted to know what I was doing. He was impressed. I told him I have converted to a plant-based diet. He felt it was working and told me to keep it up. So that was it. You can't argue with results like that. He is also younger, in his early thirties. There are a lot of people in that generation that have become vegetarian or vegan, so he wasn't surprised or judgmental.

But it is funny that he is not interested enough to find out what diet plan you are doing so he can recommend it to others who are in the same boat as you. That connection never seems to be made.

It was funny when he saw Murray. The doctor walked by Murray three times looking at him and finally recognized him on the third pass. He said, "Wow, you have lost a lot of weight." Murray told him that he was eating a plant-based, starch-centered diet, as written by Dr. McDougall. The doctor wanted to know who that was. Murray told him about Dr. McDougall and his website, but he didn't write it down or anything.

Are getting your support mainly from your husband?

Totally. I also joined four plant-based groups. Vegan Surfers is a group that explores vegan restaurants, plus, New Vegans, Plant Pure Pod, and Toronto Starch Solution. I will admit that I don't feel comfortable with any other vegan group other than Dr. McDougall's group because the food is so uncertain everywhere else. There's a lot of oil in the food. What we eat in the vegetarian community is considered the extreme end. We are way out there.

What can you do now that you couldn't do a year ago?

This is another thing. I had horrible sciatica last year. My sciatica has cleared up completely, never to return after I started this diet. I tried everything from acupuncture, chiropractor, and physiotherapy. I finally found a physiotherapist who gave me the right exercises and she did some sort of sound wave therapy. My toes actually went blue and discoloured, and I thought that was diabetes and went to the doctor. I literally couldn't sit. I couldn't stand. I couldn't walk. I couldn't sleep. The pain was constant. I am not a painkiller kind of person so I was toughing it out. My muscles atrophied. It took me until May to get my muscles back. Can I prove that the McDougall plan made it possible for me to recover? No, but I know it has. It gave me the stamina, recovery, and the general level of health that I now have.

I did so much research online about sciatica. Apparently on Dr. Greger's site, he said that there is a school of thought that little micro blood vessels that feed your spine can get clogged up with fat and that is why a lot of people have lower back pain. If you change your diet to low-fat and vegan, the pain goes away. Back pain is the number one reason why people miss work in North America. I still see the chiropractor once in a while. How can I go from having severe sciatica to not having it at all? I am sure it is my diet. But most people refuse to believe it is the cure-all for almost all the diseases.

Let's talk about your emotional, intellectual, spiritual life. Has that changed at all?

My moods are better. I am generally much happier. When my body feels better, I feel better, which makes me happy. My entire body used to ache. Now I have so much energy. It is like going back 30 years. I feel like I can work rings around other people. I am thinking clearer. Dr. Greger is saying only five percent of diseases are hereditary. It is the bad diet that is causing disease. Diseases don't run in families, diets do.

That is powerful. Dr. McDougall said this, and I thought it would

make a great t-shirt "Nine out of ten diseases are caused by eating animal products."

When you think about how the animals are nowadays, overcrowded, suffering, and sick from what they are fed now. It makes me sick to think about it. The animals are so sick and diseased and full of antibiotics. That upsets me.

What about the impact of a whole food plant-based diet on animal rights and the environment? What are your thoughts?

I have been an environmentalist, albeit, a misguided one, my whole life. I can remember in my twenties, going camping and taking an expensive biodegradable soap to wash dishes. My friends thought I was crazy. I was using this dish soap to wash dishes and my hair. People would be washing their hair with regular shampoo in the lake, and that really worried me. Oh, my God, they are using regular shampoo in the pristine lake up in Algonquin Park.

I also bought a special washing machine that was a German compact, back in the nineties and everybody wondered what it was. It is a washing machine that uses half the water. I didn't realize, in my ignorance, the impact that meat production has on water consumption and the environment until recently. Now, I have been watching some of these movies that are online. I didn't realize how bad it was. Yes, it has made me more aware of the impact of eating meat and catching fish, and the destruction to the rainforest. It has just made me more aware.

As for animal rights, what has been seen cannot be unseen. I have watched some of those horrible videos like *Earthlings* and Gary Yourofsky's speech, where they show clips from hidden cameras that were smuggled into slaughterhouses. Once you have seen that, you can't un-see it. It makes me sick that that has been going on.

We all talk intellectually about buying free range eggs. You have 10,000 chickens on the barn floor that are all squished together and that is what they call free range or free run. With the label "free run", they can be in a barn all day long, but they never go outside. However, there is an open door to the outside, but they never get to be out there. You can legally call that "free run". I was supporting that, thinking I was doing something good. Oh, these chickens are living a happy life at old McDonald's farm. At least they are not in those battery cages. I am glad that by being vegan I no longer support this terrible industry.

Have you participated in animal rights activism?

Yes, just recently. I felt physically strong enough to go on that anti-slaughterhouse march and it was wonderful. I really felt good doing that. There were about a thousand people there in downtown Toronto. I did that entire march and it was extremely hot, almost as hot as today. I am amazed at myself for doing the whole thing. At the end, we sat and listened to some speakers. I got hungry, so I walked another ten blocks to my favourite vegan restaurant called Basil Box. There you can get brown rice and tofu and you get your choice of sauces and stuff to put on it. I don't know how many miles I walked that day. It was at least ten subway stops. When I got home, I still wasn't tired. I love that I have all this energy and it is because of the starches I am eating. The old me, two years ago, could never have done this. My stamina and recovery are excellent.

I am just so excited. I have such a sense of hope, not just for myself personally but for many. I am hoping to influence more people, in my direct sphere of influence. I have hope for the world. I have hope because veganism is growing by leaps and bounds. I watched this whole report from Britain's Veg News about how veganism has gone up in Britain by 350% in the last two or three years. Imagine, and that is just Britain! It is the younger generation. When I go to a restaurant like Fresh, it's full of young people. This is what they are doing. They have seen the videos, and that disgusts them and they are not going to do as their parents have done. I have lots of hope.

The meat producers have said now if you can't beat them, join them. They are getting into producing the vegan products. It brings tears to my eyes because until you get that resistance gone, we are not going to beat them. The big corporations are too powerful. They are now buying these factories up and producing alternatives to meat because that is what the people want. I have hope for the next generation. Hopefully, they will be healthier.

I think we have had one of the most, unhealthy generations ever. The kids who grew up in the seventies with McDonald's and other junk food, with no consciousness about what they were doing to themselves, to the animals, and to the world, are the ones who are beginning to suffer the consequences with poor health. I think we were very unhealthy. The food in our school cafeteria, I can still remember the taste of it - the fake gravy, the fake beef patty and the fake potatoes. I would follow it with a Jos Louis pastry because everybody bought one for desert.

Any wish to go to Dr. McDougall's program in sunny California?

I am hoping that I will someday be able to attend this program myself, the 10-Day Program, while Dr. McDougall is still running it. I just want to go and be surrounded by fellow McDougallers. I want to meet him and I want to hear him in person.

Dr. Caldwell Esselstyn, Dr. T. Colin Campbell, Dr. John McDougall, and Dr. Michael Greger are real heroes in my eyes who are making a big difference to our planet. Campbell lost his position at the University and had one of his programs shut down. McDougall has been shunned by just about everybody and recently kicked out of a weight loss symposium, which is just ridiculous because he actually has the solution to obesity with a whole food starch-based diet. They can't market rice, beans, and potatoes, so they don't want the public to hear about the truth.

China made a commitment last week to reduce meat consumption by 50 percent. There are two billion people there!

I am sure it is mostly for health reasons because they can't support two billion sick people. Think about this. The Chinese people used to eat rice three times a day, and yet they were always slim. We blame rice and all the other carbs as the culprit for making people fat. Everyone seems to believe this common misconception that carbs make you fat.

Personally, I am not supporting the meat market anymore and I am telling everybody I can about this way of eating. Even if I help just one person, that is a worthwhile endeavour. Hopefully, that person will help one person, and then that person will help one person, and then that next person will help one person and so on. That is how we can change the world, one person at a time.

Basically, I have gotten my husband on board and I want to get my daughter on board, and by default, it will filter down to my grandchildren. If you can, influence your direct sphere by people seeing how healthy and thin you have gotten eating this way.

Do you have any goals related to your new lifestyle?

I'd like to get off all my meds. I'd like to be cured of diabetes. I want at least to maintain the levels I have already achieved. I'd like to be off my blood pressure medicine and my insulin altogether.

Did we talk about your heroes yet?

Dr. McDougall is head and shoulders above everybody else. The other most influential person has been Dr. Neal Barnard. One particular video about diabetes of his really spoke to me. Rich Roll, the marathon runner is a vegan. He and his friend did five ironman marathons in the Hawaiian Islands in seven days. He said there is no way he could have done that if he wasn't vegan. People just keep showing the power of a vegan diet. When a new vegan athlete comes along and is breaking records, it is starting to look common place.

I also just love Dr. Greger. He is a sweetheart. It's amazing to see all the information that he has put on his website nutritionfacts.org for free, and it is evidence-based nutritional science. There are no words to express how wonderful that is. I always direct people to nutritionfacts.org. Even if they don't want to change their diet but they have a specific health concern, I say go on there. It is all free and look up conditions like IBS, MS, diabetes. The latest science is all there.

I would tell new people that if you have a metabolic disorder like diabetes or a large amount of weight to lose, go directly to the McDougall Plan for Maximum Weight Loss rather than *The Starch Solution*.

I am looking forward to Dr. McDougall's new book. I have already ordered it, *The Healthiest Diet on the Planet*. I'll just give the book to people. I want to lend books to people.

I read somewhere recently that you can't talk with people about politics, religion, and food because they have such a personal and emotional investment in those things. I never thought about food. We say when you go to a party, don't talk about politics or religion with people, but we should add food to that list. People have such an attachment and visceral reaction to it. Remember, I was telling you about that guy at the pub who got angry with me. Since then, he has come up to me twice at the pub and said, "You know, I listened to what you said. I did a little bit of research into it and I am eating a lot more starches. It made sense to me and I am feeling better. I have cut out a lot of red meat and I am eating a lot more potatoes and beans, and I have more energy." Even at the last get together, he came up to me and wanted to thank me again because he was feeling so much better. He was angry at first, but he actually listened. Then, he went and confirmed the science.

That is what I have been wondering. Is it possible to get through the barrier that people have? I guess it is worth the effort if you occasionally break through.

I want to thank Dr. McDougall and his wife from the bottom of my heart, for potatoes and Mary's gravy. I can live off that, I literally could. I have lost 36 pounds and I am no longer on a downhill trajectory with my health. I am getting better, not sicker. I feel fantastic. I am full of energy and vitality. I am happy. I am thinking sharper and more clearly. I am more fit. I am a totally different person than I was a year ago. I hope I will continue to lead a healthy life. I am hopeful I won't ever be going down that road of illness and suffering ever again now that I have made these powerful lifestyle changes.

Chapter Eight
Judy

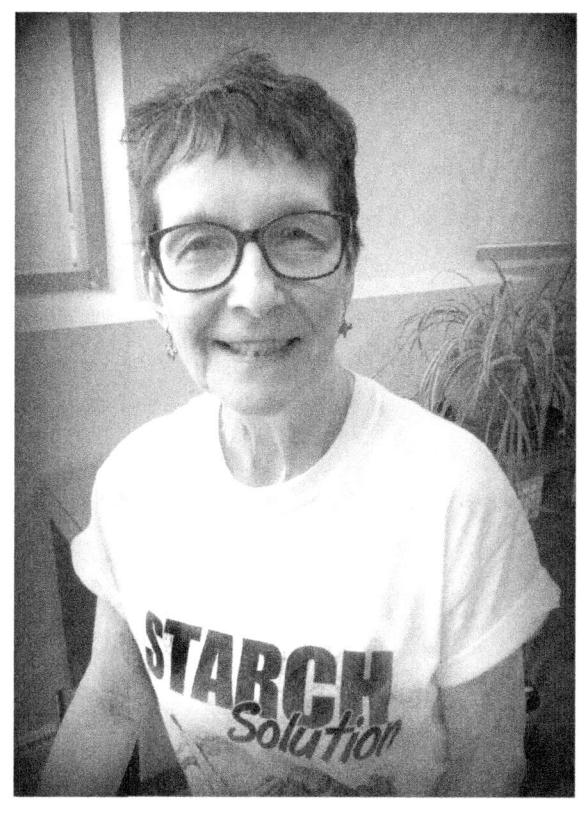

Judy didn't have a weight problem and ate what she thought was a healthy diet, but she was tired, depressed, and stressed. All medical indicators were found to be normal, including blood pressure and cholesterol. Then, in her early fifties, she had a heart attack. Read how Judy discovered Dr. McDougall's dietary program, regained her health and vitality, and has left depression, stress, and heart disease in the distant past.

Chapter Eight - Judy's Interview

Can you give us a bit of back ground information on you, your work, and your family?

I am a retired addictions counsellor and I have two adult children, one daughter-in-law and one grandchild. One of them is actively trying to follow this plan.

Can you tell us your story relative to Dr. McDougall's program? How did you get started?

I was having some digestive troubles and feeling miserable all the time. My digestive system was in such a mess. I had been tested and prescribed medication that made me feel worse and didn't really solve my problem.

Then I was cleaning out my bookcase at home and I discovered Dr. McDougall's book *Twelve Days to Dynamic Health*. I have no idea where it came from. I think the veggie fairies put it there. I ended up reading the whole book and it made perfect sense to me. I thought, "It's cheap and easy. I have all the stuff I need here in the house." I changed my way of eating and within 24 hours I could tell that all these seemingly incurable digestive troubles were going to disappear. It was as simple as that. I don't remember exactly when, but that was about 12 years ago or more.

I already had a heart attack prior to that. It was what they sometimes call a "silent" heart attack as it passed pretty well unnoticed. I had a day of overwhelming exhaustion, which the doctors told me much later was probably the heart attack. Only when my annual physical came around did I learn that there was something wrong with my heart and, as strange as it sounds, I didn't really make the connection between adopting this way of eating and heart disease.

All during the examinations and tests that I underwent in relation to my heart, nobody mentioned diet. Nobody asked me what I ate. Nobody told me what I should be eating. I was pretty slim and my numbers were all in the "acceptable" range so they probably didn't see any point. Hopefully, they would have discussed diet with me if I had high blood pressure or high cholesterol. I was pretty shocked to find out that this whole thing had happened. I felt that my body had let me down and I was very unsure about how to proceed.

When I asked the cardiologist point blank at our last appointment what I should be doing, the only advice he gave me was not to shovel snow! While my family has a terrible history of heart disease, I didn't have any of the warning signs. I thought I was eating a healthy diet but I realize now that I was not, and I was also in a very stressful work environment. I was working very long hours, spending a lot of time commuting, and eating fast, easy food when I got home and, of course, feeding that to my hapless family. Had I not changed my lifestyle when I did, I expect the heart disease would have progressed. I am very, very lucky to have found Dr. McDougall and I never forget that.

When I first started the diet, I lost so much weight, people were concerned. They thought I had cancer or something. I added back bread and healthy peanut butter, and things like that, and my weight went back up to where it normally would be.

It seems like people have too much weight or too little.

I was not overweight to begin with so when I started losing weight they just assumed I was ill.

Were you a vegetarian before you started McDougall's program?

I would say I was a borderline vegetarian. I would use a little ground chicken in a casserole, or bring home vegetarian pizza. My kids had never seen a roast, or a steak, or pork chops, or anything like that. I did eat some meat. I ate fish and skinless chicken breasts, you know, all the "right" things. At one point, I was on the Curves diet with my daughter and that was very low carb. All the meat and fish and salmon and whatever you could choke down with salads and vegetables, and no carbs at all. I don't think they advocate that anymore because it is very unhealthy. But if you eat that way, you will lose weight.

I don't understand why carbs have become so "bad" for us; they're not nine calories per gram like oil. When people hear "carbs" they think about everything from plain rice to a black forest cake. We need to differentiate between healthy complex carbs and Krispy Kreme Donuts! Potatoes are very healthy in their natural state, but not after they have been chopped up and deep fried. Low carb diets eliminate everything.

Dr. McDougall's book was on your book shelf?

Yes, he was sitting there quietly for who knows how long. I do buy books at yard sales and such places. When I saw it on the shelf I thought it was my husband's, so I asked him if I could get rid of it and he said, "I've never seen that book before."

Who else has inspired you?

After I discovered Dr. McDougall, I started reading everything I could find. Eventually I found my way to Dr. Campbell, Dr. Esselstyn, and Dr. Greger. I absolutely love Dr. Greger, Dr. Neal Barnard, Dr Fuhrman, and, of course, Dr. Klaper. I have seen many of them here in Toronto at one point or another. They are my heroes.

Do you watch YouTube? Is that where you get your inspiration from?

I do watch YouTube. I watch documentaries. I have Netflix, so I watch documentaries on there. I read a lot. I love the success stories on Dr. McDougall's website. I take my cup of tea and watch a couple of those success stories, even the ones I have seen before. I feel like I know some of those people. Cloudy Rockwell always seems like a person I would love to meet. She is from Alaska, and she managed to do this change all on her own. If she can do it there, anybody can do it. She lost an enormous amount of weight and regained her health. Her story is just so inspirational. I have watched her so many times that I feel like I know her.

This is a community. We are part of this community and it is growing in North America and around the world. Like that spud guy, "Spud Fit". Dr. McDougall is bringing him over from Australia to speak.

People from all over the world are following this diet. However they found it, people recognize that this is a healthy way of eating, and they are looking for something to change their lives. I think a lot of people are just desperate and aren't getting any help. Whatever they do, they are just getting sicker and unhappier.

Unfortunately, there is still a lot of misinformation out there. I volunteer with the Toronto Vegetarian Association, and I met a young woman who told me that she used to be a vegetarian before she moved to Canada. But, when she moved to Toronto, she had to give it up because she couldn't find a Whole Foods Market. We had a conversation about where to find actual "whole foods" rather than just a store by that name and about shopping around the perimeter of your local grocery store. You just have to go to the produce section. There is a lot of misinformation and many people believe that eating this way is very difficult. People are starting to get it. What we have been doing by eating the Standard American and Canadian diet is plainly not working. People are looking for a different solution, and our Toronto Starch Solution Meetup group can help.

How has this diet changed your life?

Well, I no longer rush from bathroom to bathroom. If you ever need to know where the bathrooms are, just call me. I used to work in a situation where I couldn't just walk away any time I needed to. I'd have to get somebody to come and replace me, and then I'd run down to the mall or the factory or wherever we happened to be that day. The first thing I did in each new location was locate the bathrooms and hope that they were close. It was making my life very difficult. My doctor was trying to help me. Eventually, she called me at home and said she knew what the problem was. She had found a parasite and she treated me for that. I may have had that parasite, but the medication I was on to get rid of it was miserable and afterwards made little or no difference. This diet has changed my entire life.

It has changed how I feel about life and the world. I am not careening towards a life of disability, the way that so many of my family members have done. I am not going to be spending 10 years on a dozen medications, just waiting to be hospitalized once again. I feel I have control of that now. I don't have to let that happen, and that is so powerful.

There is a name for taking five or more medications concurrently and it's called "polypharmacy". I find it appalling that it is so common that it has a name. According to a StatsCan report from 2015, about 30 percent of people in my age group are doing exactly that. That is where most unsuspecting adults are headed, and that just sets up a downward spiral of side effects that then need to be treated with more or different drugs. I don't believe that our bodies are meant to function so badly. We are just constantly poisoning ourselves. Most of us make sure that our cars have the right type of fuel and the right kind of oil. Our bodies are the only vehicles that really matter and we put any old kind of garbage through them, and then wonder why they break down.

What kinds of things do you like to eat? What do you eat daily?

I eat a lot of potatoes and sweet potatoes. Usually I have in my fridge either a bowl of cooked brown rice, or a bunch of cooked potatoes or sweet potatoes, or some starch that forms my foundation. Then I add to that some vegetables and beans. I do usually cook my own beans from scratch and store some of them in the freezer, but canned beans, rinsed well, are good too. I am not cooking every meal from scratch. I don't mind eating the same foods. I eat oatmeal every single morning no matter what, winter, summer, always. I'm eating steal cut oats right now. From watching Dr. Greger, I throw in cinnamon, nutmeg, goji berries, barberries, and sunflower seeds. I cook that in my Instant Pot for three minutes, and then I add ground flaxseed and hemp hearts after cooking. I usually make enough for three days at a stretch and I eat it with blueberries and black currants. My oatmeal is evolving, becoming more complex, as time goes by. When Dr. Greger talks about a new berry or spice, it usually ends up in my oatmeal. It's probably my most complicated meal except for company dinners when I get to try something a little more special than my usual leftovers, but still McDougall approved. That gives me a good chance to try out recipes that I wouldn't normally cook just for myself. Since we have started the Toronto Starch Solution potluck lunches, that's another opportunity to test and sample lots of different recipes, and I really enjoy that. The variety of absolutely delicious recipes is amazing. One of my favourite sites is fatfreevegan.com.

So, you wouldn't cook your family a slab of meat?

No, I wouldn't do that. I still make turkey at Christmas and Thanksgiving because it's traditional and they like it. But I've found as time goes by, I can't deal with a real turkey anymore so I get a frozen turkey in a box. It's already stuffed so I just have to stick it in the oven. I am coming to the point where I think I won't be able to even do that. I don't want this dead animal in my house and I certainly don't want to handle it. Poultry is particularly bad, of course, because it's very contaminated. We'll have to keep making adjustments. We've already discussed having those meals at my son's house so they can cook the turkey. We'll see.

What obstacles and difficulties have you faced being on this diet?

When I am with my extended family, they absolutely don't get it. They just do not get it. The health of people in my extended family has been so bad. My sister-in-law died from multiple chronic medical conditions last week. When she was first diagnosed with diabetes, I brought her a copy of Dr. Neal Barnard's *Program for Reversing Diabetes*. I don't think she opened it. She was so frightened because she had worked in nursing homes all her life and she knew where this condition was leading, and yet had zero interest in trying anything different. I think she was just afraid to do the wrong thing. She followed the diet the doctor gave her and lost quite a bit of weight, but still ended up on insulin. That was just the start of a cascade of medical conditions that all required treatment, usually prescriptions, which, of course, bring their own problems.

It's now a couple of years later, and she is dead. They were terrible years for her and for her family. I think she felt that the safest thing was to follow the doctor's advice. After all, what's the point of consulting all those specialists, and undergoing all those tests and procedures, and then not following their advice? She kept adding more doctors with more prescriptions, and they were telling her how well she was doing. She was very compliant with whatever they told her, and then she died. If she had read the book and followed the plan, she might still be with us. Who knows? She was six months older than I am, and I expected that we would become old ladies together. I miss her so much. Her experience has spurred my interest in helping other people avoid getting into that spiral.

What is it in the human being, that someone like you and I will do whatever it takes to find a way to improve our health. I have the pain, I am searching for the solution, yet for someone else they won't search. It's resignation. They won't try anything.

I feel that I'm taking responsibility for my health, and so are you. As a society, we've been brainwashed to think that doctors can do anything and that there is "a pill for every ill". We're led to believe that all we have to do is find the right doctor, the right treatment, and let them do their thing. If we look around among our friends and families, that's plainly not working.

I don't know whether it was because my sister-in-law worked in healthcare all her life and this was the only system she knew. You take the pills. When the pills stop working, you take the shots and you just cross your fingers and pray that you won't go blind, or have an amputation, or anything terrible like that. The idea that we could change our health outcomes by changing our diets is just so foreign.

She was very good at cutting back on quantities and she lost weight, and that helped. She lost weight by eating half a tuna sandwich on white bread instead of a whole one. She didn't change the food itself, instead she lost weight by depriving herself. According to her paradigm, she was taking full responsibility by following the instructions of all her doctors as well as she could. Occasionally, their advice was conflicting and it was up to her to try to make sense of it. She had a very bad time of it. When your specialists start complaining about treatments prescribed by your other specialists, you know you are in trouble! She looked like she was 100 years old when she died. Yes, she was diabetic and she got medication instead of good lifestyle advice. Yes, her heart was enlarged because she was diabetic and on lots of medication and that leads to heart damage. And yes, her kidneys were shutting down, but none of that is a natural consequence of being 68 years old. Everyone dies of something, but you shouldn't die of everything. She had everything in the end.

It is something about how the medical institution wields such power. The medical doctors are on the "God pedestal". What the doctor says goes, in most people's minds. Except, the doctors have little to no education in nutrition.

When I meet someone new and they tell me they have a medical condition, I make a habit of asking whether they have been talked to about their diet. Typically, they have not or if they have, it's of the "half a tuna sandwich on white bread" variety. Through doing this, I've come to realize once people have a diagnosis, it is very hard for them to change. My sister-in-law was seeing a well-known specialist, and the well-known specialist said this is what you should do. By the end of her life, she was seeing at least three different specialists, for three different chronic conditions, and having nurses come to the house a couple of times every day to check on her meds and change her dressings. She was getting the best that medical care has to offer. Each time she went to see them, they would say to her, your numbers are great. You're doing well. Your blood sugars are terrific, you are losing weight, your blood pressure is good, yada yada, and then she died. It is very hard to go against three specialists and say, "I am going to start eating this new way instead of listening to you because what you are doing isn't helping."

I'm sure it would be easier for us to change our lifestyle to prevent disease but it has become part of our culture to just keep doing the same thing until we get a diagnosis, and then deal with that. Our healthcare system is, in reality, just a disease management system, and it's not even very good at doing that.

Any flack from your kids or your husband?

Not really. They don't complain really. If they want to eat meat or dairy, they have to get it and prepare it themselves.

Nobody is criticizing or poking fun at you?

My son teases me a bit occasionally but it's all in fun. When they were little, I used to bake greens into cookies, make brownies with carob, and that sort of thing. They like to kid about how badly they were treated, having to eat that food. Now, they are good sports about it. I feel that I'm doing this for them, as much as for myself, because I don't want them to have to watch me deteriorate like that and have to worry all the time about me. I want to live well and then drop dead one day, out hiking or doing something else that's enjoyable.

Any obstacles or problems with friends?

No, not really. Some of them probably think I'm a complete whackadoodle but that's okay. I find it very interesting that some people feel they need to give me dietary advice when I say I eat this way, but those same people wouldn't dream of challenging anyone who walked in with takeout from McDonald's or KFC. There is often someone asking where I get my protein, or my calcium, or even my fat, but I've never heard anyone with a takeout container being asked where they get their greens. That's bizarre, if you think about it.

How about your doctor? Is he on board? Does he get it?

I have a woman doctor and I'm very happy with her. I think she may feel that what I'm doing is risky but she checks everything, including my B_{12} whenever I go for my physical, and everything is fine. She doesn't criticize me but she's not encouraging either. I suspect that if I ever do have a medical crisis, she may point to my way of eating. I like her very much and she has been my doctor for over twenty years. She's been through all this stuff with me.

I am off all the medications that the cardiologist automatically put me on. There were three medications because that is probably what the protocol says, and a lifetime of low dose aspirin. I am off those things and my doctor helped me do that safely. I also consulted a pharmacist about how to stop them because I am cautious about things like that. I didn't go back to consult the cardiologist. It would have been a waste of his time. I found it interesting that the pharmacist looked up the best process and the effects of getting off my beta blocker. Of course, that's a very good thing to do but I wondered how many times she had ever been asked about how to get off some of these meds. Most people probably don't even realize that's possible because they are never given the option. Many of the chronic conditions people have are just routinely treated with a lifetime of meds.

My beta blocker has a list of over 30 possible side effects and some of them are quite severe. At the time of finding out about the heart attack, I was so stunned and I didn't have all this information yet. It never occurred to me to question what the cardiologist told me to do. I was still in that place where I thought they had all the knowledge.

I wanted to go to cardiac rehab because I was afraid to exercise on my own, and so he referred me, although he didn't seem to think it was really warranted. A young doctor there found that my blood pressure was too low to work out so we phoned the cardiologist. He took me off one of the meds after just a couple of weeks. If I hadn't gone to rehab, who knows what might have happened to me. I had already taken a week off work to adjust to feeling so ill from the meds. When I actually had the heart attack, I didn't miss any work at all because I didn't realize it had happened, and didn't feel any long-term effects. How crazy is that?

You haven't had another heart incident in over 12 years. What do they attribute that to I wonder?

Good luck and genes, probably.

Where are you getting your support from?

From Dr. McDougall's website, until we managed to start this Toronto Starch Solution Meetup group. Now and then I would post a message on McDougall's message board, hoping to find somebody local. There are always messages cropping up about support groups in San Francisco or somewhere. I thought there must be somebody else in Toronto. I can't be the only one in a city this size. Eventually I got a response from Kathy. We arranged to meet at Whole Foods Market at Yonge and Sheppard. We had a cup of tea. Kathy and I continued posting and Judith met us for tea. When we got to around six or seven people, Judith offered to host a potluck in her home, and we thought that was wonderful. It was so nice to sit down with all these people, all this lovely food and people you don't have to explain yourself to. Where do you get your protein? You need fat, you know? It was so nice and we really just bonded.

Then, we thought we should become a meetup group because nobody wanted to do that in their home naturally enough - to invite the world to your home for lunch. We started having them at my church. Now, anybody who wants to come can come. We've got lots of room and lots of dishes, and it has been just great. The potluck lunch is growing steadily and some of our members are branching out doing different things, like Tom and Petra having picnics in the west end. They have also hooked up with Plant Pure Nation. Some of us had a potluck picnic at the Toronto Veg Fest because so much of the food there has oil or something else that we don't want to eat. I was wearing a Starch Solution t-shirt and several people approached me to say that they had read the book or to ask questions about what we do.

I really enjoy volunteering with the Toronto Vegetarian Association even though they don't advocate this particular way of eating. They don't tell people what to eat and what not to eat aside from meat and hopefully all animal products. They are doing really good work and I enjoy the people I meet there. It's encouraging to go to the Total Health Show, or the Yoga Show, and meet so many people who are looking for ways to be healthy. They are not necessarily on the same path that I am on, but they are all really interested in a healthier way to live and in helping the planet. For me, that counterbalances the people I see in the grocery store with a cart full of "edible food-like substances" and animal products.

How do you personally problem solve at parties, dinners, wedding and social events?

Anywhere you go, there is nearly always a salad and some kind of vegetable. Our church has a weekend retreat every winter in February and I request the vegan option. It was always imitation chicken breasts. I started writing on the comment cards, asking if we could just have real food like beans and rice. Last year, they did it and it was wonderful. They put a big section in the salad bar with different kinds of cooked beans, grains, seeds, and lots of lovely greens. I was able to make my own meal and one of the organizing committee members asked if they could photograph my plate as an example of the wonderful food we were eating. Of course, I was one of the very few people actually eating that food.

When I go to a wedding, I eat a little bit of whatever is there, if it's remotely appropriate. I think that one day isn't going to change my life. As I read somewhere recently, it's not so much what we eat on the 15 days a year that are special occasions. It's what we eat on the other 350 days that makes the difference. From day to day, I am much more careful about it. I always go towards making the best choice that's available, although I confess I have a weakness for sweets and sometimes pay the price for that.

Do you carry food with you?

Usually when I go out for the day alone, I carry a couple of baked potatoes or some whole fruit or something with me. Choices are limited for healthy food and, if I get really hungry, bad things could happen. I usually take something with me that won't go bad, not rice. Spoiled rice can do very nasty things.

Do you have any advice for beginners who are just starting out on the McDougall diet?

If I were advising someone who was just getting into this, I would say read a lot, go on the website, watch the videos, immerse yourself in this. Read recipes and figure out how we cook without that ubiquitous "tablespoon of olive oil" that starts every recipe. Then, clean out your kitchen and restock with McDougall friendly foods. I think if people try to dive in immediately, without being prepared and informed, then the temptation will come up to order a pizza, just this once at the end of a long day, and then you keep feeding your addictions and don't get to really see the results.

Do you have to plan ahead?

Just in the very beginning. Take an extra week or whatever it takes to learn and understand what you are doing and why it's important, and then prepare yourself. Get rid of all your junk food and go out and do a decent shop. Figure out how you are going to cook beans or decide whether you are going to use canned beans. Canned beans are fine. I have a lot of frozen food in my fridge and I don't buy canned vegetables but I certainly buy frozen vegetables. Prepare yourself so you don't get caught off guard. When I come home from a long day, I don't want to have to think about what to eat and start cooking rice or beans from scratch. It's important to plan ahead to protect ourselves from temptation. If there was junk food in my home, at some point, I would end up eating it. Of course, there is no reason to have junk food unless someone plans to eat it. Just saying! It's important to switch the focus away from what I am giving up to what I am getting. What I can get from this lifestyle is amazing.

One thing for me was learning to keep it simple. Some of the recipes are really complicated. Even after all this time, I come across recipes with ingredients I've never heard of! Keep it simple and you don't drive yourself nuts. If you like to cook, as I do, then on special occasions it's fun to try something more elaborate.

For myself, day to day, I keep it simple. Beans and rice, or potatoes or sweet potatoes and vegetables, and a bowl of vegetable soup and some fruit, and that's how I eat. If somebody's coming over, then I make something a bit fancier. I do like to cook, but I don't do that three times a day for myself.

We are so indoctrinated with this food system that they call SAD (Standard American Diet) that when you ask somebody what they had for dinner last night, they will name the meat - chicken. Is that all you had? Steak, and nothing else? They don't mention the other things on their plate. So, when you suggest to someone that they give up meat they think they are going to starve! We've probably all had people look at us with terror in their eyes when we suggest cutting out meat and dairy. It's a big change to get rid of that chicken and try to picture something else when you haven't really been aware of eating other foods.

In my family growing up, we always had vegetables but they were really for decoration. It would be a spoonful of mixed peas and carrots and maybe some instant mashed potatoes to fill the empty spaces around the meat course. It requires some preparation to change that mindset. I remember when I quit smoking many years ago. For about six months, I smoked one or two cigarettes a week that I got from a friend. The idea of giving up those last couple was terrifying to me, like letting go of my lifeline. I can completely understand people's fear of changing their lifestyle in this way.

Has this way of eating impacted your mood, or your attitude?

I have been given to depression my whole life to the point where sometimes I couldn't get out of bed in the mornings. Dr. McDougall talks about limiting sleep as a treatment for depression and I think there is truth in that. I could sleep for days when I was really down. I can't imagine getting to that state again. It just doesn't happen. Part of the change is that I feel empowered to take care of myself. I eat well, exercise every day, and sleep normal amounts of time. Even though I am retired and have become an "empty nester", I feel like I have a goal in life and that certainly is helpful.

What about energy? Did you notice a difference?

I don't remember being aware of lack of energy except when I was really depressed. I think I just always felt I had to keep going. I do remember one time when I mentioned to a new doctor that I was feeling tired and had no energy and she said, "You are almost 45, you know." After that appointment, I looked for a different doctor and never saw her again. There seemed no point. What would she say to me if I was 75?

So maybe it was actually low energy. I had kids, a house and a full-time job. Maybe I was low in energy, but I had reason to feel tired. Now, I have loads of energy. I sleep like a log. I wake up early. Every morning, I am raring to go. I feel good all the time. Literally, all the time, unless there is some normal crisis of life like a death, but day to day, I feel great.

Do you notice any difference in your clarity or your ability to think?

I was extremely stressed when I was starting this diet. Stress has so many effects on your body. It can make you foggy and unable to think. I am much clearer now.

There has been a lot said about the impact of a whole food plant based diet on the environment and animal rights. What are your thoughts?

Well, interestingly, I find the longer I am at this, the harder it is for me to watch people eat meat and not say anything about it. You have to divide your mind if you eat meat. I remember as a small child that moment that comes to all of us, realizing that this chicken used to be alive. I had never really known that. I remember as a little girl, one day realizing that this was a dead body on my plate. It was like a crisis in my life.

I read somewhere one of the doctors talking about how all children have that realization and how your family gets you over it. You have to eat meat or they make fun of you or pressure you until you move past that. We all have to compartmentalize, you know. I love my dog. I love my cat. I love my cockatiel, but I am eating this chicken. I remember actually before I became vegetarian feeling guilty because I had a cockatiel flying around the house and I was eating chicken. I actually remember wondering, "Does he know I am eating a bird?"

The truth was that I knew and that made me very uncomfortable. I was sitting across the table from a little girl recently. She looked at the roast chicken on the middle of the table, and she said, "That's gross". She looked over at me and I agreed. That was probably her moment of realization.

I would never murder my dog. But, for many years, I supported people murdering other animals that are every bit as intelligent, every bit as terrified. The longer I am away from eating meat, the more I am able to let those thoughts in. I read somewhere just recently that every meat meal begins with that animal begging for their life. Just think about that.

I don't walk down the meat aisle anymore. I'll go around the other three sides of the store before I walk down the meat aisle. There is an Asian market that I like to go to that has one of those big aquariums. You know, you pick out your fish and we'll kill it for you. I never could deal with lobster, ever. But the idea that people can come along and say, kill that one, feels just awful to me. I am becoming much more extreme in that way.

Animal agriculture has a huge negative impact on the environment and it would be one of the easiest ways to make a big improvement in a short time. We are running out of time and this is really low hanging fruit in the climate change field. The more people that make the change, the better off we will be and it is starting to happen.

Consumption of some meats is going down but it has to be a grassroots movement. Corporations are so powerful, and they fight every change that anyone tries to make towards legislation that could help us.

When we were at the Remedy Food Event a few weeks ago, one of the speakers was talking about when she became vegan and started explaining to people. She said one of her friends was so angry and she said she was going to go and buy meat and throw it away. It is just irrational, almost hatred - because you say you are not eating meat anymore. Food is very emotional. We associate food with celebrations and love. You celebrate your victories, successes, and your parents, and everything is all about food. It's an irrational attachment.

We see a lot of hate stuff on websites when people talk about going vegan. It is incredible the responses that people have. Nobody is telling you that you have to do it. Go read something else. It is that "roll your eyes" attitude at veganism that is kind of bizarre. What does it matter to other people what I eat? The reaction can be really, really powerful.

I never put two and two together that I was eating an animal that was alive a few days ago. I didn't get it until I was 60 years old. I never put the two together because they put the meat in neatly wrapped styrofoam packages. The meat industry is a master at hiding the truth from us and distracting us from what is really going on.

You are absolutely right. Very few of us ever see meat in its bloody, gory natural state. By the time we get it, it's easy to forget where it came from. My best childhood friend lived on a farm and they took a pig to the butcher. I was staying with her at the time and was probably in my early teens. Her dad carried in half a pig cut right down the middle from nose to tail and laid it on the kitchen table and we spent the rest of the afternoon cutting it up into roasts and chops. They could save money by doing that part themselves. I didn't know whether to cry or throw up. I had been eating pork my whole life. I just had never seen it like that before. I've never forgotten that experience and I sometimes wonder what must happen to the psyche of people who work in slaughterhouses. Talk about compartmentalizing.

How do you see yourself changing the world or contributing to this movement?

For me, it's just one person at a time. I am so happy that we have this Toronto Starch Solution Meetup group because we each bring our super powers. What I have to offer is access to this space and these facilities at my church. Other people have really good social media skills, really good speaking and writing skills, and lots of creative ideas. We all bring our super powers together and we can do so much more organizing and publicizing than any of us could do alone. I think if I can just get one person to look at this and pay attention then that is the greatest thing. When one influential person in a group like my church congregation gets on board, they can influence others. This way of eating is consistent with the ideals of the Unitarian Church. We follow seven principles and the seventh principle is "Respect for the interdependent web of all existence of which we are a part." I feel very positive about this whole experience as it is not only healthy for me, but it aligns with my personal values. Little by little, we'll spread this message of wellness.

Are you planning on doing anything new?

I liked giving a presentation about Dr. John McDougall and *The Starch Solution*. I would like to expand it to other Unitarian Congregations in Toronto or other groups.

Have you converted anybody into a whole food plant-based diet? How does it make you feel when someone listens to you and follows your advice?

I've converted just a couple of people. I am so happy because, generally, the people you have the most influence over are the people you see most often. My family are just dropping dead one after another, it seems. I don't want to lose everyone who is important to me so if I can get some of them to change, that's good.

A few people here at the church are losing a couple of pounds per week eating as much as they want. Why hasn't everybody in the world jumped on this band wagon? Here is the secret. You can be healthy, and look good, and it costs you nothing.

What do you think it is? The media? Tradition?

I think it is all those things. The media keeps us so confused. Once a week, there is something new. Oh, it's not fat, it's sugar. Never eat this. Always eat that. There is always something on the internet with the title *Five Vegetables You Should Never Eat*. What are those? I think people get so confused, they say, "Oh the hell with it. It makes no difference. I'll eat whatever I want." Everybody is sick and everybody is fat and society is beginning to think this is normal. It is normal to be 55 and be headed down the road of being disabled by heart disease, cancer, diabetes, arthritis, Alzheimer's, and dementia.

Do you have hope for the future of our planet?

I do. It's hard but I do. That is why I keep reading and looking at all these documentaries. There are a lot of people out there who get it and are trying to do something about it and now we are doing our thing to try to do something about it. I have to keep reminding myself of all those people who are all on the same page.

You know, when you are in the grocery store, I often think that I'd like to do a little game show. You line up all the shopping carts over there, and the people over here, and see if you can match them up. The stuff that people have in their shopping carts is just unbelievable and they wonder why they are 40 pounds overweight and diabetic. I checked out recently behind a senior-looking couple, and in their overflowing cart the only food-like item I could see was a loaf of bread. They had boxes of snack cakes, bags of chips, 2-litre bottles of pop, cases of bottled water, lots of sugary cereal, and one loaf of bread. Look at what you are eating. I often see people studying labels in the store aisles, but they are checking which highly processed edible food-like-substance has the lowest levels of sodium or sugar. Nobody has told them that those things aren't food.

There is a lack of the right information. I watched a documentary recently about childhood obesity in the United States, and parents were trying to deal with it by buying all these low-fat cookies and low-fat potato chips and low-fat this and low-fat that. It is not good food. It is not healthy. It is just high sugar, low nutrient junk. They are so conscientiously going down the aisle, reading all the ingredients and getting all the low-fat stuff. It is still cookies. It is still potato chips.

Why is that so difficult to understand?

Well, I think it has to do with the fact that sugar, high salt, and fatty foods are actually addictive. Opiates are being distributed through those foods. The parents don't want to give it up either and some of them even say that. They don't want to give up the chips and pop because they are addicted too. Life can be kind of grim and a bag of chips makes you feel better. I can relate to that. When I was young, I can only remember knowing three people who would be considered obese.

What we think of now as junk food wasn't available yet, but you could get pop and chips and pies, cakes and ice cream and candy. In our family, we had ginger ale when we were sick and pop, occasionally, as a treat. Drive-in restaurants were just starting to appear and, of course, that opened up another whole range of possibilities. We went there on Saturday nights as teenagers, but not once or twice every day, the way some people do now. Back then, cars came equipped with cigarette lighters and ashtrays, front and back, but not with cup holders. Then, they started making handy little cup holders that you could buy and hang off your door. Now, we get standard cup holders front and back, and can buy empty calories everywhere and consume them all day long, but most of us would probably be astonished if our new car came with ashtrays.

What is it that makes you go and research and try to find out the cause? Why do you do that and everyone else has every joint in their body replaced? Jane Fonda had all four done. Two knees and two hips, and she is a health fanatic. Nobody ever told her about John McDougall, and she lives in California too, just up the road from him. I don't know, and that is the big question.

I don't know how all these wonderful lifestyle medicine doctors have kept going all these years. There they are, trying for decades to give us the secret of life, and it's free. All we have to do is use it. Dr McDougall was dis-invited from the Obesity Medicine Conference last spring. He was probably the only one who had a real workable answer to obesity, and the answer is free! How these doctors have managed to hang in there for all these years is amazing to me. Dr. Campbell's son talks about growing up all his life, seeing his father being maligned, made fun of, criticized, and losing his courses. Yet, he is still at it and he still wants to tell people because he has got the truth and the science to back the truth. All that professional ridicule - can you imagine living through that? Yet, they keep on.

Thank goodness they do. What I find fascinating is that we all have the same heroes. The same five guys and chef AJ. We are all YouTube junkies and we all watch the weekly John McDougall webinar. They're our heroes and they're the people I want to listen to repeatedly.

I do watch them over and over again. You know Dr. Greger's annual summary video. I watch that over and over. There is so much information in there. How could I have been alive for 67 years and not know these things? As they say, there is no money to be made from giving people the solution to their problems that doesn't require medical intervention.

I have been recommending this book about the pharmaceutical industry to people. It is called *Deadly Medicines and Organized Crime: How Big Pharma Has Corrupted Healthcare* by Peter C. Gotzsche. It's available in the public library. It is appalling what people do to other people. The author is comparing the pharmaceutical people to the mob, how they operate in very similar ways. They bribe people and they lie. The author has all these inside emails that he gained access to. They just try to get in there and make a billion dollars before they get caught. Then, they release things on the market that haven't been properly tested or that they know have bad effects. By the time they get caught and nailed down, they will have made a billion dollars. Then, they get fined some relatively insignificant amount, and then they start on the next one.

This is completely crooked. They falsify the test results and cherry pick people to put in their studies. If you aren't doing very well in the beginning, they kick you out of the study because they only want the "good" people in there who will show the results they want. He says they don't sell drugs, they sell promises about the drugs. They always talk about the wonderful results you are going to have.

Those ads that run on American TV, show people dancing or cycling, barbecuing, playing with their kids, and then they mention some of the risks, like sudden cardiac arrest, internal bleeding, kidney failure, etc., but, not to worry, because your erectile dysfunction will be rectified. Imagine if you went to buy any other product that you can think of and it came with warnings like that. Nobody in their right mind would buy that. But with pharmaceuticals, somehow, we just overlook those warnings and forge ahead.

One of the possible dangers of stopping my beta blocker was that it could cause me to have a heart attack. I was prescribed it in the first place because I had a heart attack. In what universe does it make sense to put something like that in my body every day for the remainder of my life? "Adverse drug reactions", as they call them, kill more than 100,000 people a year in America. If a car manufacturer or some other company started knocking off 100,000 people every year, there would be a problem. Not so for Big Pharma.

You are not on any meds anymore?

I am on Synthroid because I had my thyroid removed. I don't know if I would do that again, given the choice, but it's done now.

Is there anything that we have left undone?

I don't think so. You have been very thorough. I am surprised that we had so much to talk about. I always think that my story is one of the simple ones.

Are you kidding? Having a heart attack, and then finding Dr. McDougall's book on your book shelf! We'll see each other when we are in our nineties.

Yeah, we'll still be here coming to this group.

Chapter Nine
Jane

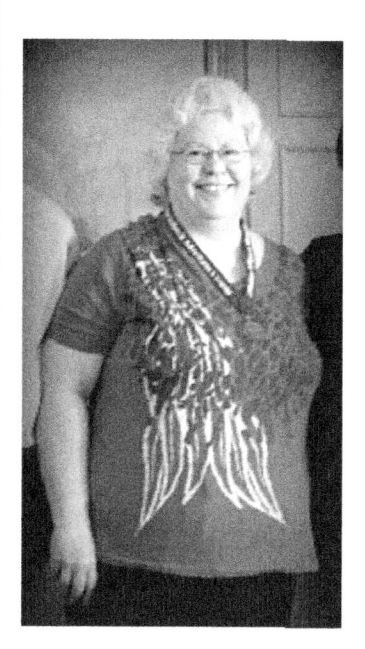

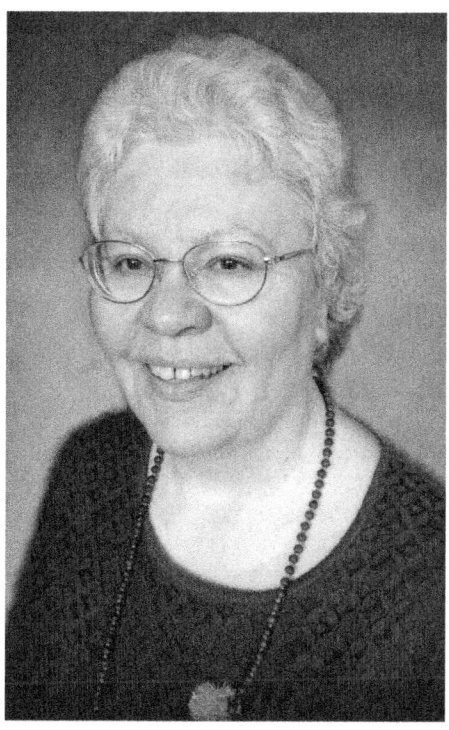

Jane was struggling with stress and depression. She also suffered from various aches and pains, and had a fatty liver. Every time she tried a new diet, she was destined to fail. It wasn't until she discovered Dr. McDougall, that she was finally able to get her weight under control. She has lost 65 pounds so far, and improved a number of health issues.

Toronto Starch Solution Meetup Group
Group Toronto Starch Solution Meetup

Chapter Nine - Jane's Interview

Tell me about your background, and your upbringing.

I was born in Guelph. My father was a high school teacher, and we moved to Lindsay, so I grew up mostly in Lindsay. When I was in grade seven, we moved out of town to the country, about five miles from Lindsay. When I finished high school, I moved to Toronto. I was 17 and I lived on my own. I got married when I was 18. I was married for four years, and I've been in and out of Toronto ever since.

How did you come to Dr. McDougall's program?

My doctor told my parents that I was far too small, I was only six pounds at birth. My grandmother told me that my father used to stuff me until I cried. I don't remember that. I've never remembered it in any therapy that I've done. But, by the time I was a year old, I was too fat. I was put on skim milk. For my entire childhood, I was fat. The very first time I ever went on a diet was at age 12. I decided I was only going to eat three oranges a day at lunchtime. I did that for a whole week. I used to walk around the house, trying to get thin. This is what I did at 12, with no knowledge and no understanding. I got kind of faint by the end of the week and that was the end of my first diet. I've been on so many diets. I did the Stillman Water diet in my twenties. I did the original Atkins diet, which didn't even allow fruit and vegetables. You were only allowed lettuce, can you imagine?

I was married at the time. My ex-husband had a bit of a weight problem, and we did this diet for two years. We worked at the race track at that time, so when the horses went to Fort Erie we had to follow the horses. We'd go by all the fruit stands and our tongues were practically down on the road, we wanted fruit so badly. But the mind prevailed, and we resisted. I think it was the beginning of the end of our marriage, because it does terrible things to you when you eat meat, eggs, cheese, and a little bit of lettuce, and you live on that for two years. It was dreadful, when I think of it now. My doctor at the time said that my blood levels were way too high, and I scoffed at it. I didn't know of any health problems that I had. Of course, I was only twenty. I said no, it says this in the book, so this must be the way to go. I don't remember why I stopped the diet. I think maybe by then, my ex-husband and I split up. But it's amazing how you get an idea in your head and it overrides your intuition, it overrides all your senses. Everything in you is crying out for something different but you don't listen to it. You do this thing that you're damned determined you're going to do.

My ex-husband actually did lose weight on it. I never did. Maybe I lost 10 pounds. But in two years, I never lost more than those 10 pounds. All I could say is I could eat as much as I wanted and I'd never gain weight. But I never lost weight. I think I did a lot of kidney damage to myself although I didn't know that at the time. So, I went off that diet, and over the years I followed other diets. Needless to say, I always had a weight problem.

I did the Fat Flush diet by Ann Louise Gittleman in 2006. It was the easiest diet I ever did in my life. It was simple, and I lost 65 pounds in six months. But as the months went on, I got very sick. My diaphragm, just below my rib cage, got so tight, as if someone had a steal cord that they had pulled as tight as they could possibly tie it and squeeze it even more. I couldn't lay in bed because it was so painful for me to put weight on this extreme tightness. I slept in a chair and I used a collar to protect my neck. I had a collar from when I suffered whiplash years ago. I'd wear the collar, and that's the only way I could sleep. It got to the point where I could hardly breathe. So, I went off the diet. I couldn't understand why everyone else could do this diet and they could lose 150 lbs and it would work for them. They'd all be nice and trim and look like models. It didn't work for me. I just got so ill. Of course, as soon as I went off the diet, the weight came back on so fast.

It was impossibly fast. How do you put on 50 pounds in a couple of weeks! Okay, I'm exaggerating a bit. But, you know, all the weight I lost was put right back on, and then some, of course. So that was really disheartening.

Then, I read the *Carb Sensitivity Program*, which was written by a naturopath, Natasha Turner, who's in Toronto. She's quite well known; she's been on the Dr. Oz show. She has a whole slew of naturopaths working in her office. She writes in great detail about insulin resistance. I highlighted stuff, and underlined stuff, and cross-referenced stuff. I read every single line in that book. I even researched some more articles that Natasha Turner recommended, because I wanted to know a little bit more about kidney issues she had mentioned, but there wasn't a lot of information about it in the book.

When I went to a naturopath in her clinic, they were all doing the same program. I tried that diet for a week and I was so sick. I just couldn't do it. I felt dreadful. Now, I have to say, I had hepatitis from one of my trips to India. My liver was very badly damaged from that. I don't handle fat well anyway because of the liver damage. There's a lot of food I became sensitive to. I could eat certain foods before I had hepatitis. After having hepatitis, I could not eat those foods. Maybe, that's why I get so sick on these diets. Other people with stronger livers, they don't seem to experience symptoms like I do. Anyway, I did notice something with the naturopath I saw at Natasha Turner's clinic. Her nose was covered in oil, and she was a young woman. I thought that was very telling. She was not handling it, even though she was nice and trim.

I just said to myself, that's it, no more low carb stuff. I'd had enough of that, it's not going to work. I'd just end up getting sick, so I accepted being fat. One of the things that's probably important - I did a meditation practice in the mornings so I didn't have time to prepare breakfast at home. I would go to a Golden Griddle, near Yonge and Eglinton, every day for breakfast - every single day. That was the way I could do the meditation practice. If I went out for breakfast, I had enough time. I'd eat three-egg omelettes every day. When I changed jobs, (I was then in Yorkville) I'd go to Flo's Diner and I'd have three-egg omelettes every day. I've probably eaten more eggs than anyone you know. I did this for at least 15, if not 20, years. I have a feeling my tight diaphragm is related to the eggs. That's my feeling. I can't substantiate it but I think that's what it is.

I got blood work done in 2015, and it was really quite alarming. My urate levels were very high, where they were putting warnings on the lab reports. It was high enough that I could have had gout, but I didn't, not yet, anyway. Cholesterol was too high. I had a fatty liver. I had an enlarged spleen. My CRP (C-Reactive Protein, an indicator of inflammation) markers were way too high. That was a warning on the report, and my ESR (Erythrocyte Sedimentation Rate - a measure for inflammation) was way too high.

I knew back in November of last year that I needed to do something. I'd been sitting on the fence for years. I had tried to do low carb and macrobiotics, but I just couldn't keep it up. I had totally bought into this insulin resistance thing. I was sold. That was the reason I was fat. I thought, these markers are terrible, I've got to do something about it. I decided to try, once again, to do the low carb diet. This time I did Jon Gabriel's diet, which is a little less restrictive than Atkins, and you know, he's such a nice guy and he has such a positive spin on everything. He uses self-hypnosis and all kinds of things, and it works like a dream for all of his people.

I was determined I was going to do this, and I tried over the weekend. By the time, I was ready to go to work on Monday I could barely lift my legs. I just couldn't lift my legs. It was unbelievable. But what did I do? I didn't go out for breakfast that day, but I went out for lunch and had eggs. I could not lift my legs. Well, okay, that's just not going to work. To hell with it, it's not going to work. I hummed and hawed about macrobiotics and low carb because how the heck was I going to be able to do this. I can't do the low carb but I've got bad insulin resistance so what was I going to do.

I pulled out a book of John McDougall's that was sitting on my shelf. I had rejected this a few years back because I had boiled potatoes and yams for breakfast and sprinkled them with vinegar. By the time, I got to work I had lost my voice completely. It wasn't just a little bit, it was completely gone. I thought, well, I can't do that. Instead of just investigating further and realizing that maybe it was due to the vinegar, I just dumped the whole concept.

I thought, well, I've got to do something, so I pulled out John McDougall's book again. I started this diet properly on January 17th of 2016. At first, I was still putting almonds on my cereal. When I got salads from Freshii, I would still use avocado and tofu. I didn't give that up for at least the first three weeks to a month, and I still lost weight. I lost a great deal of weight right away. Then slowly, slowly, I stopped the tofu, I stopped the avocado, I stopped the almonds. I got cleaner in my approach to the diet. Eventually, I stopped eating breakfast cereal because I heard that it would be better if you didn't.

I've lost 65 pounds to date. All my blood markers have gotten better. The urate went down, the cholesterol went down, triglycerides went down, HDL and LDL went down. The non-HDL cholesterol went down. Fatty liver is gone. My spleen is less enlarged, it was 14.4, now it's 13.3. CRP went from 12.4 to 9. These results occurred after 16 weeks on the diet. I did not get a diaphragm problem, not the same as it was. I can now move my legs quite freely and easily.

Would you say that you've got health issues that have resolved or are resolving?

Yes, I have health issues that are resolving. The ability to move my legs has improved a tremendous amount. My flexibility, like turning and twisting in the shower, is much better. When I used to have to bend over to pick something up, I thought my head would explode. There was so much pressure in my head. Now, I don't have that at all. My arms are more flexible, I have more flexibility to put my arms behind my back. It's so much better than before because I could barely do it at all.

Are you noticing changes in your job performance?

In some ways, things that used to seem like an enormous burden of a chore, is less of a chore. There's always something that you don't like to do, and it's less of a challenge now to get through that. Yes, resistance is less.

How have you dealt with your family and co-workers with this new way of eating?

Nobody seems to be too concerned. Everybody's willing to let me eat this way, it's not a big problem.

Do you get curious questions?

Not much. Everybody notices, I think 65 pounds is hard to ignore. But very few people have asked me about it. A couple of my co-workers have said, "Yay! Good for you!" They're good about it, but I'm surprised how many people haven't asked me more. But maybe they think they couldn't, or they shouldn't. Or, they're shy about it. Who knows?

Do you think that will change when you lose another 50 pounds?

Oh, for sure, I'll get more questions then. Because I'm still large, I still have weight to lose. For many people, being more than 30 pounds overweight is still way, way, way too fat, especially with young people, if they're trim. It's just part of the culture.

Has your family been behaving differently towards since they're seeing you're smaller now?

I don't see my family often. Nobody lives in Toronto but me. My sister is deceased, but I see my brother-in-law and niece about three to four times per year. They've noticed, but don't comment very much.

I'm sorry to hear about your sister's passing, did she die of a chronic illness?

She had kidney cancer. It wasn't diagnosed for a long time; she had all kinds of symptoms. It was at the time of SARS, and so the specialists were so worried about people coming in to hospitals and potentially being exposed to SARS. So, unfortunately, it affected her care.

Do you ever wonder if things would have turned out differently for your sister if she had known of this way of eating? I'm thinking of T. Colin Campbell's research showing how animal foods turn on cancer cells, and how plant-based diets turn off cancer growth.

I am absolutely sure if she had come to this diet she wouldn't have died. I am not so sure though, if she would have been open to it. It's hard to know. It's unfortunate.

In your own personal life, are there any difficulties or obstacles that you have faced or are facing now with following this way of eating?

The hardest thing is going out socially in restaurants. That is probably the only problem. With a lot of my friends – that's what we do – we go out for breakfast, lunch, or dinner, and that's how we meet up, how we socialize. Or, we go out for afternoon tea. I have found a couple of restaurants that will prepare food without oil for me. It's a bit restrictive for my friends, who like to be very liberal with their eating. That's the big entertainment part, to do the dining out thing. It would be great if there were more restaurants that would prepare food without oil.

Are your friends concerned about the way you're eating? Do they ever wonder if it might not be the healthiest thing for you?

A couple of my friends that I see very rarely, my friend Jane and her husband –he's studied a lot of literature, and he's convinced, totally sold on the "You must have protein at every meal" thing. That's probably the biggest thing that people are sold on these days - how important protein is.

At work, they have professional development, and then they have personal development programs every year. They bring in a dietitian and anybody can join. It's very thorough. They meet up for several months in a row and they get lots and lots of information on diets. But the dietitian is saying, "You've got to have protein at every meal." So, because of this getting drummed into people, they just can't imagine going vegan - even though grains, legumes, and potatoes are all rich in protein.

I remember my co-workers were so thrilled with the dietitian. She was very generous with her information. They're all thrilled about it, just thrilled. I think they were trying to convince me to go along. Well, I'm sorry, I think it's kind of contrary to just about everything the doctors I'm following say. None of them have lost weight, and I have. I don't mean to gloat, but, they just didn't have success losing weight, and yet, they still buy into it. It's like Dr. McDougall says, "Everybody loves good news about their bad habits."

Do you think that by you doing what you're doing, you are leading by example?

That's the only thing I think I can do. I have to prove it because people are so convinced that starches or carbs are bad. People go to this wonderful Indian restaurant in Yorkville, and they'll have the chicken makhani, which is the butter chicken, and they'll have the littlest bit of rice and eat just the meat because they're controlling their carbs, you know. But they're all trying to do the right thing, because they've all been sold on this. The only way that I can stand up in front of someone is "Well, I eat 80 to 90 percent, maybe even more, of carbs, three times a day, and my health is getting better." But until I get down to what's considered an ideal weight, nobody is going to be sold.

How's your doctor feeling about this way of eating?

She's into alternative therapies. She herself does juice fasting a few times a year. If a naturopath wants any blood work done, or any tests done, she's totally willing to go along with what a naturopath asks. So, she does seem to have a very real belief that diet makes an impact. I don't know that she's sold on vegan, though. But she is willing to see what the results show. She was very worried about the levels of my CRP and the uric acid. She was very happy to see them go down. I think she's willing to be convinced.

Do you feel like there's a bit of pressure on you to show how well this works? Or are you okay, do you feel very relaxed and certain that this is the way to go?

I am very happy with it. It's totally liveable. I don't have to say even that it's a diet. Because it's so simple and I feel totally satisfied with the food. I don't feel like I'm depriving myself. Sometimes, I would like to have some chocolate. I know that I can have some chocolate when I'm not trying to lose weight, but if I want to continue losing weight, I have to avoid it for a little while.

Where is your support coming from?

At the beginning, the biggest support was watching all the McDougall YouTube videos. That was so helpful. When I'd get weak, and I'd think, oh, I'm not getting enough results, I'm not feeling that strong.

It's been very helpful to have it reinforced many times over by the scientific experts and the doctors. Watching films like *Forks over Knives*, *Plant Pure Nation*, *Cowspiracy*, and others has been inspirational. I watched a lot of Caldwell Esselstyn as well, which is very supportive. His explanation of why it is important to avoid oil is very helpful. It's great. The nice thing is so many doctors are following this now. I keep hearing about more and more doctors that are doing very close to this program, if not exactly like it. I think there's at least 15 to 20, and they're all well-known doctors that are making presentations around the country. I'm very happy about that. Even those mini-videos from Dr. McDougall are extremely helpful.

The books themselves are impressive and have made a big difference for me. I have them right by my living room chair. Sometimes, I'll open them up and I'll look at the before and after pictures in *The Starch Solution*. When you've been overweight so long, basically 61 years for me, it just seems impossible that I could ever be thin. For everyone else it will work, but it will not work for me, you know. I've had that experience too many times. When I'm feeling so satisfied from the food, and I step on the scale and my God, I've lost two pounds, how lucky is that! Oh, I'm so glad! It's working, wow!

It's very motivating to read about the Star McDougallers with a similar weight problem. There's a woman on there who was 150 pounds overweight. Her story shows you don't have to lose three to four pounds per week. She lost one pound per week on average, and she ended up losing a tremendous amount of weight.

Now, of course, there's the Toronto Starch Solution Meetup group, which is really helping me. There are other people going through the same thing I am. They're eating the same food I am. They're having the same problem in restaurants that I am. So, you're not in total isolation.

Are there others, besides Dr. McDougall, who have inspired you?

I've read *The China Study* from front to back, and I loved it. I've watched some of Dr. Greger's YouTube videos, and Dr. Doug Lisle – his explanations are very helpful. I've listened to them a few times. Jeff Novick, I love Jeff Novick, I think he's marvelous. His calorie density DVD is to die for. I want someone to make a new documentary, just on calorie density. I'd like it to be done in a factual way, not just copying a presentation.

If they could put the correct information about insulin resistance since there's a big flaw in insulin resistance education. That flaw is that you turn sugar into fat. That is so wrong. What happens is you eat fat and the fat is stored. The sugar is not stored as fat, it's the fat that is stored as fat. That is the biggest mistake in the whole insulin resistance thing. Here I am, when I first started this diet, thinking I can't put ketchup on my potatoes because it'll just turn into fat - the belief that I have to have absolutely zero sugar, as well as eating really plain starches. But it's okay, I can have ketchup with my potatoes because it's the fat, not the sugar, that is causing insulin resistance. That is so useful for me. I'm living proof that it works.

There are several Star McDougallers who were extremely heavy. There's a man who was 450 pounds, and he's lost 250 pounds. That's someone who is living on 80 to 90 percent or more carbs all day long. You tell me if it's working. It's working, here they are. This is typical. If people keep eating this way, and it's a very satisfying and delicious way to eat, you get good energy and you lose weight. These are people who are able to eat this way and keep their weight off for the rest of their lives.

Do you have any advice for beginners?

I would say, get some education. Make sure you know what you're doing. If you're not a reader, watch the YouTube videos. If you can do both, do both. Read *The Starch Solution*, read Dr. Esselstyn's book, Prevent and Reverse Heart Disease. Read *The McDougall Program for Maximum Weight Loss* by Dr. McDougall. I would tell them to get some decent recipe books but not to be stuck on recipes. If they like really simple food, don't worry about trying to make complicated recipes. Some people would rather have baked potatoes all the time than eat brown rice. Nobody said you have to have brown rice, quinoa, and barley all day. Eat the food you really like, whether it's brown rice or potatoes.

It is a bit misleading if you get a book like Plant Strong, for example, which is a nice cookbook, but there's loads of nuts, and nut butters. If I tried to eat that way, I would never lose any weight. If people are worried about protein and calcium, they have to read *The Starch Solution*, and *The China Study* by Dr. T. Colin Campbell. For me, it's been an interesting journey, and I've really enjoyed doing all this research, but not a lot of people do.

What do you feel you can do now, that you couldn't do before you started Dr. McDougall's program?

Aside from a lot more flexibility in my body, it has opened more doors for me. I'm looking forward to getting into a plane seat without having to have a double-seat belt, getting into a train seat and being able to use the little tray that you have there. I'm hoping that my feet will improve after losing more weight, so that I can walk a lot easier. Then, I'll be able to travel to India again.

Considering physical, as well as emotional and intellectual effects from eating this way, would you say this has had a big impact on your life?

The biggest impact is that I no longer live in fear of my cancer returning. I was diagnosed with cancer of the uterus in 2010, and while surgery took care of that, I was still concerned that the cancer would come back in another place in my body. Now, I know that eating this way will prevent any further cancer from occurring.

There's a lot said about the impact of a vegan lifestyle on the environment and animal rights, what are your thoughts?

When I look at it from a world perspective, I think that nobody on this earth needs to be hungry, even in Toronto. There's so much green space where people could grow vegetables. It's amazing how prolific the earth is. We're not very smart in some ways. We could do so much more. I'm really hoping that the people who believe in eating meat will not be so incensed by the growing movement towards plant-based food that it will get violent or criminal. I think a lot of people will resist it tremendously, and I think it's scary. I've heard in the Amazon forest, people have been murdered for resisting the deforestation to allow for more cows to eat. But I think the world will be a more peaceful place if people were more plant-based. I think people are calmer in their attitude when they eat a plant-based diet. It's more natural for people. People will be less ill, not only physically, but a lot less mentally ill if they're eating a lot more vegetables. I really am a big believer that a plant-based diet is the way to go. It will save the world. It'll save people from starving to death. It'll improve people's health. It will help the environment. I thought the film, *Cowspiracy*, was so revealing. What a fantastic documentary that is. Hopefully, it will have a tremendous impact on getting people to pay attention to what is happening to our planet when billions of people are eating meat and dairy.

How do you see yourself changing the world?

I don't know if it's a big impact, but I do believe I am making a difference in a small way. When I get down to a normal size, I'll be a walking advertisement then, and that will have impact. I'm not eating any meat, and that helps to decrease the use of animal products, which helps the world. Perhaps considering we're all one consciousness, this has an impact. Every change we make will influence our environment, even if it's a small thing, because that will have ripple effects. My goal is to be a Star McDougaller. I hope my before and after pictures will be inspiring to others, and hopefully, they'll change their diet and lifestyle because of that.

I'm so grateful to Dr. McDougall, hammering out his message year after year after year, and doing those 10-day programs, several times a year. I'm telling you, if I hadn't read his book, I'd still be on the fence. Macrobiotics? Low-carb? Macrobiotics? Low-carb? I'd probably have had a heart attack, or a stroke. Or my cancer would have come back somewhere else in my body, and who knows where I would be now? I hope Dr. McDougall keeps going for quite awhile longer. He is such a dynamo, and he's now educating younger doctors to continue his work. I'm very impressed with that.

Is there anything else you think is important to share that hasn't been talked about?

I want people to know I've had my gallbladder out, and I am still losing weight on this diet. A lot of people think when you've got no gallbladder, you're doomed. You're going to be fat for the rest of your life. I'm proof that is not true.

With being overweight, you feel like you're ostracized or judged, and that is a fact. You certainly are overlooked or judged as slothful or stupid or slow - for some reason, our society thinks that fat people don't have any brains. I think a lot of things are sold because the person looks good. The salesperson sells himself, and that sells the product. I think that when I lose weight, more doors will open for me.

When I ride the subway, I see so many more people, young people, who are very large, larger than I was at a young age. I think that this information is so needed now because young people are beating themselves up. Young people have bought into believing they have no discipline, or they just didn't try hard enough – all that kind of self-abuse that you do. Not to mention all the people who will help you abuse yourself.

They're doing a sugar tax in Britain. Making sugar more expensive is not going to help these people if they've got loads of fat in their meals. I suffered so much myself from judgments, being a heavy person, that I always feel bad when I see people who are even fatter than I am. I have so much empathy for them because I know how much they go through. It's so important, this education. People do not have to go through this. It's an easy solution.

With people who don't want to give up the meat, do you think there could be an addiction component?

When I separated from my ex-husband, back in 1977, I had an uncle who was very radical, and he was a vegetarian. He'd just shove his beliefs about what to eat down your throat, at any opportunity he could. People rolled their eyes and just ignored him, but he was so far ahead of his time. I was rather distraught over my separation from my ex-husband, and I was going to be moving to Scotland. My uncle had come over to visit my parents. Once again, he went on and on about the evils of eating flesh. I was very impressionable at that time as I was so emotionally upset over the whole thing with my ex-husband. My uncle made such a big impression on me, even though I'd never listened to him before. I was just as much a meat eater as anybody else. I thought, maybe that's why my marriage didn't work, it was all the meat. I decided I was going to be vegetarian as soon as I got to Scotland. I got a job at a university there – I was a table maid, and I was a vegetarian. Of course, what did I eat? I ate loads of cheese and I ate loads of eggs. But I'll tell you, I craved meat like crazy. My God, for a whole year, it was insane how much I craved meat. Now, I don't care, but it took awhile for it to get out of my system.

By 1988, I was eating chicken and fish, in addition to all those eggs and cheese. Now, I don't crave it at all because I don't eat the fat and oil, and I believe that helps to keep the cravings at bay. I will say, for those who think we need fats, while still having so much fat on our bodies, we probably won't be deficient in fats for quite awhile.

Thank you, Jane, it's been a pleasure to interview you today.

I've really enjoyed speaking with you, and I hope my story will help at least one person.

Chapter Ten
Carol

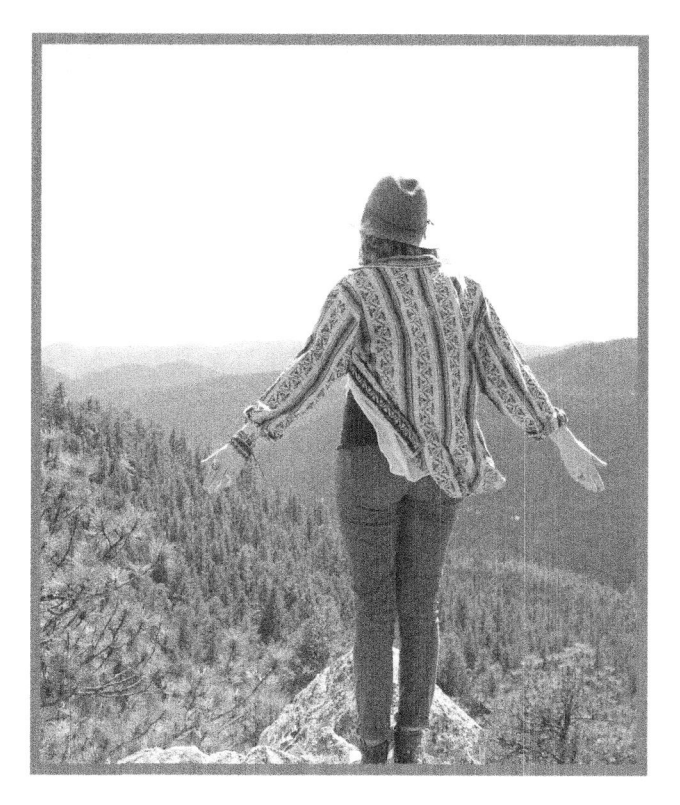

Like so many others, Carol was slowly gaining too much weight and then the unthinkable happened. Carol was diagnosed with breast cancer and Parkinson's Disease. Her daughter told her of this doctor in California who was having amazing results at reversing serious illnesses with a starch-based diet. Carol and her entire family flew to California for Dr. McDougall's 10-day program. Find out about Carol's incredible weight loss and health results after following Dr. McDougall's program for 18 months.

Toronto Starch Solution Meetup Group
Group Toronto Starch Solution Meetup

Chapter Ten - Carol's Interview

Please tell us your story, relative to Dr. McDougall's program, *The Starch Solution*.

I had always dieted. I've gone through everything; Bernstein, Weight Watchers, Jenny Craig. I'd say that I'm a yo-yo dieter; lose the weight, then gain it back plus more. As the years went by, I kept putting weight on, and then more weight on, and then I got sick. I developed breast cancer. I had gone to the doctors to check on the tremor in my finger. They did the physical and sent me for a mammogram, and called me back for an ultrasound, which is typical, because one of my breasts has always got a lump in it. It turned out it was the other breast and it was cancer. It was 3.5 centimetres. I had seen the doctor on Tuesday, saw the surgeon on Wednesday, and the next Tuesday, I had a mastectomy. My daughter Amy, who has always encouraged us not to drink milk or eat dairy, advised us to also give up the meat. That's what precipitated me going to see Dr. McDougall. My health was in bad shape.

I found out I had Parkinson's. I was going through chemo and radiation. I was just exhausted. I thought, well, we'll go to Dr. McDougall's 10-Day Live-In Program in California. The title of my story with my kids is "It was a health inheritance." It's a lot of money to go to Dr. McDougall, but it's well worth it. We went as a family - myself, my husband, and our three grown children. I said to my children, this is your health inheritance. When they were growing up, I worked full time. They got fast food and boxed food from No Frills,

Sobeys, IGA, whatever it was. I felt I did a bad job in raising them food wise.

I went to see Dr. McDougall due to Amy's constant information on what's best to eat. She herself was struggling with doing it, and because she was struggling we said, yes, yes, okay. When we moved back to Burlington, we had to stay at Amy's house for three weeks while we waited for our new home to be ready for us to move in. She put Dan, my husband, on Dr. Fuhrman's plan, GBOMBS – which is greens, beans, onions, mushrooms, berries, and seeds. Dan's diabetic and by eating that way his blood sugar went down to normal. He was doing very well. Amy made fabulous dishes, and it kept her going too, because you had to make them for someone other than just yourself. When we moved into our new home, it was difficult to continue without Amy's wonderful cooking. Dan would just put cans of beans together without any seasoning and eat a bowl of beans, to keep his sugar down. Well, that got boring, not exciting, and so we went off. We're junk food eaters, there's no question about it. We love our snacks, and we love salt and oil and sugar. We gained more weight. Amy still encouraged us – she said, "You did so well, you have to keep this up." At first, until you get it, you don't realize how much you're killing yourself.

For Dr. McDougall's 10-Day Live-In Program, I knew we both had to go, otherwise, we'd never learn it unless we did it together. I thought Dan was going to flake out after the first day and say I'm not going to do this anymore. But by the third day he said, "I can do this. This is great." He did very well. He went off four of his nine medications. I dropped my cholesterol down 40 points within the 10 days. We felt so much better, and we got used to eating the food. We chose not to use salt. Therefore, it was strange to us to take out salt, oil, and have minimal amounts of sugar intake and eat whole foods. We got to the point where we liked it so much that any time we went off the plan, we thought, "Oh, I don't like this." When we got back home, we got into making our own food. We like it better, and it's more flavorful for us.

That's why we got started, for health reasons. Dan's diabetic, I have to get my body clean. After my mastectomy, I had four months of chemo, then radiation. I had to wait a year to get my second mastectomy. After the second surgery, it took a minimum of six months to get over the exhaustion. My body was in shock. When I went to McDougall's I was just starting to feel, not normal, but better. That program escalated my body to feeling better, eating the whole food, plant-based foods. It just went on from there. People were saying my mind was clearer.

You've mentioned a number of health issues. Do you have health issues that were resolved or are resolving?

I have Parkinson's, and that won't get resolved by food. That's just the way it is. What I can do is slow it down. I've also been diagnosed with osteoporosis, and I have to admit it put me into a depression for a week. No question about it. I thought I'm going to be walking down the street, and I'm going to fall down and I'm going to break something. That's when I thought, "What's the point of eating healthy if this is going to happen."

I thought, well, I can do it with food. I didn't want to take anymore pills. I try to drink almond milk every day, but just in case I miss, I take 1000 mg of calcium, 500 mg in the morning, and 500 mg at night. I make porridge with almond milk and I put extra almond milk in it. That's how I make sure I get my calcium because I don't eat regularly enough of the calcium type foods, I know that. I will confess that the Parkinson's diagnosis was the start of me going downhill on this plan. We were doing very well, like honestly, we were almost perfect. After the diagnosis I thought, what's the point, I'm going to have a big piece of apple pie and ice cream, buttered shrimp and all that kind of stuff that I love. But after a bit, we stopped and went back on the plan, which was great. We feel so much better.

The osteoporosis can be a result of the medication you're taking. Do you think things will improve once you are done with the anti-estrogen medication?

The anti-estrogen drug I'm taking causes trigger finger, and a whole bunch of stuff, but it also depletes your bone mass. I have to have the anti-estrogen, just to make sure the cancer doesn't come back within the next five years. But I have to make sure I get enough calcium. I'll be on the anti-estrogen drug for another year and a bit. I've got tingling and numbness in my hands and feet, that's all part and parcel with the drug. So when that goes, hopefully it won't be a permanent thing. Even though I wish I didn't have to take it, I don't want to take the chance that I will have another recurrence of cancer. If I eat healthy, as Dr. McDougall says, you don't have to have cancer. If you're eating whole foods your body has the ability to fight it off. I wish I'd done this when I was 35, and stuck with it. But, that's the way it is, and you know we're enjoying life now so I can't complain.

Have you looked into the work by T. Colin Campbell, who has shown how eating whole food, plant-based will turn off cancer growth?

Well, that's what Dr. McDougall said. The 10-Day program was filled with lectures and all kinds of information. Dr. Klaper, he was one of my favorite ones there because he would just talk straight, and I could click with what he was saying. You kind of think, I should have eaten better, but I didn't, so I'm not going to blame myself.

The past is the past. What matters is today, what you choose to do today. You do things the best you can, and if eventually the best you can do is to stay committed to this 100 percent, then that's amazing. I don't miss meat. It is the salt, the oil, and the sugar. If I could stay away from the sugar, I think I could stay away from everything.

I think those three things change our brain chemistry, and they just drive us to want more of those foods.

Oh yes. Like, literally at night you're going, Dan, you have to get me some chips. It's an addiction. It's a physiological addiction. It's said it's a worse addiction than heroin or cocaine, partly because they're so accessible, these foods. They're everywhere. You just walk down the street and there they are. They're at the corner store, in the snack vending machines, and they're on TV. We're constantly being shown those foods. In society, there are no restrictions to eating those foods. In the world we live in, it's not a negative. We know it's bad, but it's not illegal.

We touched on Dr. Campbell, and you mentioned Dr. Klaper. Other than Dr. McDougall, who else has inspired you?

Amy, my daughter, is a big inspiration. She really is the spearhead of all this. She is determined to make us as healthy as possible. I admire her for that, because it's hard when people roll their eyes at you. As soon as you say you are vegan, or whole food plant-based, they just think, "I don't want to talk to them. They're weirdos." It's true. That's the way it is. With our whole family going to the McDougall program, we could eat together all the same foods. It was wonderful that I didn't have to cook special foods. For example, Amy has to cook separate meals for her kids, and things like that, especially one of them because he doesn't eat anything. For our family potlucks, we could get together and everybody brings a McDougall dish. It's all whole food, plant-based. Amy's the leading inspiration. And she's done so well.

She's special, your daughter.

Yes, that's true. All my kids are good, you know, really good. Kate, she's so funny – she makes the best recipes. She tries out different things: tortierre with lentils, and it's delicious.

When did everything start for you?

2012 is when I discovered I had cancer and Parkinson's. The journey for dieting has been since I was 13. When I learned about Dr. McDougall from Amy, I thought I can't do it on my own because Dan will sabotage me. If he isn't on it, he won't know what I'm doing and so he won't eat this food. I said, "Yes, your Dad will go." Then, Amy calls me up and says Kate wants to go. And I said, "Okay, I'll take Kate." Well, Dan said, "You have to take Brian. You can't take two of the kids and not the third one." We took all three of them. It was a great experience. I would do the 10-day again, to tell you the truth. I really would. The knowledge is amazing, and the people you meet are all there for a specific reason. You can see them getting better throughout the week. That's very inspiring.

How has your life changed, given everything that you've done up until this point?

I feel better, and I feel more knowledgeable. I feel like I can control this. There's no reason why I can't do this. I like that I'm not getting wrong information. I don't have to eat like Dr. Atkins – all meat – because you knew that was wrong, but you tried it all anyway. Hey, you get to eat butter and bacon, why not? Weight Watchers is a good one, there's no question about it, but there's still the fat content and you have to watch what you're eating. With Dr. McDougall, it's a much easier way of eating. Whole food, plant-based eating is easy. There's no question about it. You can have potatoes until you're blue in the face. You can have rice. We love starch. We made up a whole bunch of different recipes for these things, and followed recipes too. It's the easiest food plan you can do. You don't have to think too much – what I made today I threw together, and it was delicious.

You've mentioned the difficulties you've faced with your health, and in trying to "stick" to this way of eating. What kinds of obstacles do you face?

You know, when I leave the house, if I stay on the plan, it's not hard. If we go out to eat, we can eat at Wendy's and have a baked potato and salad. We can go to the Pita Pit and have all vegetables with mustard as a no-oil dressing. We can eat there without any problem. When we go to a restaurant, we can say a salad but with no meat or cheese or anything, so it's very doable. But after I have a drink, it's not very doable.

I have a glass of wine, and I find I relax more. So, socializing makes it more difficult for me. If I have that glass of alcohol, it's like the flood gates open. I want chicken wings, I want French fries, you know. I have to really watch it. We've travelled a lot. When you travel a lot, and you're eating out, it's hard to get people to understand that this is what you want. They don't get that. Some places don't even let you do that. It's easier since we bought a trailer. When we travel I take our Instant Pot and our Vitamix, and we make our own food.

When we go to people's places for dinner, I feel bad for them. They say, "Oh, what can I cook for you?" I say, "We will bring our own food." I don't want them to feel obligated to make food that they wouldn't like. Your taste buds have to adjust to this food, to whole food. It's delicious food, and it tastes so much better, but your taste buds have to adjust. People are always asking us about it, and we try not to say too much because we get very excited about it, as you know. It's amazing what it can do for you. A family member had us over for dinner last Thursday and she said, "I'm making all the foods you can eat." I said, "You don't have to do that, we'll bring our own food." She said, "No, no, I want to." She made everything we could eat and it was delicious. And they ate it! It was great.

When you are out visiting family and friends, what kinds of issues usually come up?

At first, people thought, they'll never stick to it. People think that when you're on a diet, you know. I find that's amazing that people would pooh-pooh it so quickly because it's just whole food. Or you get people that are very interested, but don't want to have anything to do with it because once you say no oil, well…. They can do no meat, or less meat, but they want their eggs, and they want their yogurt. Those are the challenges you come up against. I don't want to talk about it with them because you do it all or nothing. That's the bottom line. You do it all or nothing. You can't have a piece of meat and expect your arteries to stay clean. You can't have oil; you can't have French fries without building up plaque. That's what Dr. Klaper was saying. That's what I always remembered, and that's what kept me on it. He showed a video with the actual blood cell, and the plaque building up. He explained it so simply. That's what I need. I don't need all the medical jargon. I need simple language and visual aids.

Is your doctor supportive of the McDougall plan?

Oh, she's so on board with this. I gave her *The Starch Solution* book, and she's reading it. She says she tells a lot of her patients about it and what's happened. I brought her in some food once. I made a pumpkin spiced oatmeal dish. She ate it right there! She said, "This is delicious! I can have this every day?" Her questions were, "What about my sandwich? Without butter what do I put on my sandwich?" I said, "Put avocado – it's high in fat but it's better for you. Or you can make some tofu type spread, or use crushed tomatoes." She said, "What about cheese?" I said, "Well, no, because it's dairy." She's doing as much as she can, and she's a very healthy looking woman. She's very, very, good and I'm glad I've got her as a doctor. She really wants this to work for me, and for other patients. I know that the dairy industry has their claws in deep with the doctors with the whole calcium issue. Then, of course, there are doctors who have bought into the whole protein thing. I'm really lucky my doctor is open to whole food, plant-based eating.

When you go to parties, weddings, special events and other occasions, how do you problem solve?

It really is mind over matter for me. If I say, I'm not going to do it, and I do not do it, then I don't miss it. I can manage the whole evening, and I don't feel deprived. I feel in control. The best thing to do is to try and stay in control because it makes me feel better. At the end of the evening when I go home, I don't say, "Oh, I shouldn't have done that." No regrets. For me, it's mind over matter.

You had talked about how alcohol affects your ability to make good choices. If you're at an event and you have a drink or two, even if you have said to yourself before, I'm not going to do it, is it still a struggle for you?

Not if I've made up my mind. When I go in there iffy, or uncomfortable, and have a glass a wine, that's when I can get into trouble. Now, it doesn't happen all the time. Don't get me wrong. It's not like if I have a drink, then I eat everything in sight. But I've noticed that my resolve is weaker if I have a drink. Sometimes, a drink helps to relax me a little more, and if I haven't made up my mind before to not eat, then I may be a little more loosey-goosey about things. I may get into the dip and crackers, and other appetizers, you know.

Do you have any advice for beginners?

I'm not sure if I have advice. I do recommend they start it gradually. You gradually develop a palate for it. According to Dr. McDougall, he recommends you cut out dairy first because that's one of the worst things. If you have to cut out something, cut out dairy. Once you're used to being off dairy, then cut out your meat. Next would be to cut out the oil. You can make your potatoes in the oven instead of frying them. You can make your rice full of flavour. We put everything in it. I don't eat vegetables, I wouldn't have a bowl of broccoli or cauliflower like some people, but they go into all our chili and stews, and it's all delicious. Experiment as much as you can with a lot of seasonings and spices, especially hot stuff. We really like hot stuff now. We've developed a palate for it, and we never used to like it. Now, oooh, I can put that sriracha sauce on there!

Do you find if you put in a lot of spice, especially the heat, you don't need the salt?

That's right, that's exactly it. I don't cook with salt, because Dr.

McDougall advised us to not cook with salt, but I do add it after. Thank goodness for the cooking lessons we got at Dr. McDougall's because they showed us how to cook like a lot of different chefs. I have a non- stick pan. I don't cook with oil, instead I use water. It never sticks at the bottom, it's fabulous. The Instant Pot, I like it so much. You know I bought two of them, and also a separate liner. I don't use anything else now. A lot of dishes can be ready in 20 minutes. I put a squash on, and it's only three minutes for this type of squash to be done. You can have your food ready within an hour easily, and have five or six dishes. It is readily available if you plan, meaning you have the food in your house. You just keep up with the shopping, and have the knowledge on how to prepare it.

What can you do now that you couldn't do before starting the McDougall plan?

I can think about what I'm putting in my body because I know the science behind it. That's why I like the McDougall plan. When I had tried to lose weight in the past, I would often go on some fad diet, and I'm not saying Weight Watchers is a fad diet, but I didn't understand the chemistry of food, how it affected all the cells in your body. Now, I'm more informed. That's what I can do now. I can be more informed, have more knowledge, and understand why this works better.

How has this way of eating impacted your mood, your quality of life, your energy, attitude, all of that?

My mood is great and I sleep like a baby, and I'll share that I have a history of not being a good sleeper.

Do you feel overall, you'd never go back to how things were before?

No, never. The goal is to continue with whole food, plant-based eating. That's the goal. That's a goal we will continue for life. For Dan, with his diabetes, he must keep eating this way. For his age, he doesn't have high blood pressure, so he's healthy. We must keep healthy. I mean, there's just no bottom line.

Do you notice a shift in how your mind works? Do you have more

clarity of thought, or a better ability to grasp complex issues?

I notice it. After chemo, you have "chemo brain", or "chemo fog" they call it. But it lasts longer than you think. I do notice that with this way of eating, I have much clearer thinking. Now, I don't know if it was because my chemo fog was very bad, and I couldn't remember words. I would think of something, but some other word would come out. However, on this plan I don't have that problem anymore. There's no question in my mind that I've improved. I feel a difference; my friends have seen a difference, a big difference.

Do you think by eating this way your recovery's been a lot better?

Yes, I do. I can feel my body healing itself when I'm eating properly. I can actually feel it. This is helping the cells get better. This is helping my liver to not absorb all these toxins. It's just cleaning out. I can feel it. I can physiologically feel that it's working. I do. It's like I have this self-awareness now. I recall when I first began to eat this way, I had some interesting digestive changes. At Dr. McDougall's for the first three days, I didn't have a bowel movement. I thought, oh, this is not going to work for me because you feel terribly uncomfortable. They said, "Don't worry, it'll happen." Of course, it did. I've never had such major bowel movements in my life. Now, I have three or four a day. I can wake up in the middle of the night and go to the bathroom. It's unbelievable, so the food really keeps your body clean. It really makes a huge difference. I should say we have a lot of flatulence. We don't care. We walk along the street, we don't care anymore. If we're with friends we just say, "Don't walk behind us." Better to come out that end, you know.

There's been a lot said about the impact of a whole food, plant-based diet, or vegan lifestyle, on the environment and for animal rights. What are your thoughts?

I honestly never cared about the animals. I figured they're raised to feed us. That's what humans do. I never had that vegetarian/vegan empathy. I went to see Dr. McDougall, and I still didn't have any concerns for anyone but me. It was about me, it wasn't about the animals. It was about my health. Then, I came home and I watched *Forks over Knives* and *Vegucated*, and we saw some stuff at Dr. McDougall's. Then I realized how horribly the animals were treated. I realized how poorly they fed them, and the overcrowding is so bad that they're eating each other's feces, and then they're pumped with antibiotics and hormones.

The realization was I was eating all of that. It wasn't just that I was eating the meat, I was eating their crap, and chemicals. Then, I found I was more empathetic. I never would hunt or kill anybody, or fish because I think that's cruel. But getting it from the supermarket, I never worried about it, I never thought about it. To tell the truth, I was not an animal activist. Then, after doing this, when I think about eating meat I think about the actual whole animal. If I see a piece of meat or someone shovelling down some stuff, I can see the animal. I can see the lamb. I can see the pig. I can see the chicken. They're ugly birds, but still, they're alive. They've got a life. I have more empathy now. There's no question about it, but at first, I didn't go in there saying I'm doing this to save the animals.

Do you have any further goals related to diet and exercise?

I do need to exercise more. With this beautiful weather, we take the dog out every morning for a 40-minute walk. We have a gym downstairs. My goal is to use the gym on a regular basis, not just the hot tub and the steam room, which I go down and use about three times a week. I have to do that because I need to get my joints moving. I need everything working better. I know I'm not going to run a marathon. I'd love to learn to surf. We're going zip-lining in the spring, and I want to be in good shape for that. The walking is the most important thing, and I'm doing it every day. If the weather's bad, I can go into the mall. Our dog is a service dog, so I can take him with me.

It's said that even doing a daily 40-minute walk, especially for us older folks, can make all the difference in the world. It can stave off issues with dementia, arthritis, and so on and so forth. You don't have to pound your feet by running. I watched a program, with a Dr. Norman Doidge, and it was on neuroplasticity. It was different studies on different diseases that people had. The reason I watched is it started with one with Parkinson's. I had read about it and I wanted to hear what this guy did. This gentleman in Australia who had Parkinson's and was on medication for Parkinson's, walked his way away from medication. He walked 75 minutes every other day, and he doesn't have to take medication. He's just unbelievable. That's what I can say, that's my goal, to stave off Parkinson medication as long as possible.

This is a big question, but I think for all of us who switch to a plant-based way of eating, it does have a ripple effect. How do you see yourself changing the world?

When you ask that question I think of my daughter, Amy, who is very involved with the Toronto Starch Solution meetup group and she loves it. I shared with her that I was thinking I might post a whole food, plant-based dinner in the paper, and have six people come out and have a free meal. I'd like to do it on a regular basis. Maybe once a month, and get six different people each time. I could hold cooking demonstrations. We can meet and talk about eating a starch-based diet, and watch a movie while everything's cooking. I think that's something that would be very interesting in Burlington. I think we'd get a lot of action.

I know how to market and organize events. I don't mind having people over for dinner. My doctor says, "I want to come over to your house for dinner." I'll invite her over. You know, that kind of thing.

What about your life goals? We all have life goals at whatever age we are.

I'd like to live with good mobility. That's my life goal, to stay as mobile as possible. My main life goal is to stay committed to whole food, plant-based eating, to tell you the truth.

Have you "converted" anyone in your life to this way of eating?

I think we've converted some people to eating less meat. I don't think we've converted them not to eat eggs or have a bit of cheese. But they see the impact it has on us. It's that leading by example thing.

Is there anything else that you feel is important to share that hasn't been talked about in this interview?

I want to share how pleased I am that I've found this solution. That's it. I've found this solution for a healthy lifestyle that lets me eat starch, which I love, and there's no reason for not sticking with this plan. It's good food. As I've said, my logo with my family is that it was a "health inheritance". I'm sure they would have liked the money instead, some of them, but you know, we gave them a health inheritance.

That's the best inheritance of all.

It's priceless, and no one can steal it from you. You'll never lose it, you'll never run out of it.

Chapter Eleven

Dan

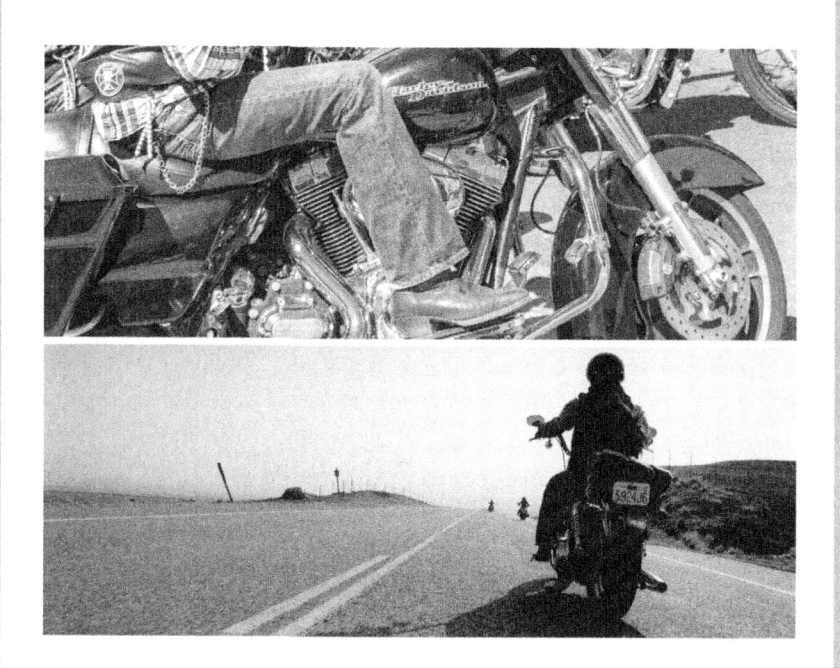

This retired police officer was suffering from obesity and diabetes. Dan knew he had to make some drastic lifestyle changes if he wanted to get his life back. After following the McDougall lifestyle for 18 months now, Dan has lost over 100 pounds, is off most of his medications, and is enjoying life to the fullest. He is travelling the world with his wife, and riding his Harley Davidson.

Chapter Eleven - Dan's Interview

Can you give us a little bit of your personal history?

I was a police officer from 1974 to about mid-2005, and then I left the public sector and went into the private sector. I was the vice-president of an investigations company out of London, Ontario. I've got three children, two daughters and a son. We've had a good marriage. We've travelled a lot and we've been married 45 years now.

I have always battled with my weight. Since my childhood, I had been heavy. I grew up with the notion that I was overweight and that is just the way it was going to be. My mom was a great cook. My dad was a good cook, too. We always had lots to eat. When my wife first met me she had never been to a family dinner where there were so many desserts. My mom would make pies and cakes and tarts, and my dad would always come in with his specialty butter tarts. You know, nice big butter tarts, just full of that sweet gooey syrup you get in a butter tart. When I joined the police department in 1974, I weighed 202 pounds and during that period of 33 years, I got up as high as 279 pounds. It was a battle. When I left the police department I weighed in at 237 pounds.

We found out I had diabetes when I was in my mid-fifties. My one daughter, Amy, was always concerned about this. She said we have got to do something about that. About four and half years ago, she had been doing a lot of reading about Dr. Fuhrman. He had a plan. We had moved from Port Stanley back to Burlington. Our place wasn't ready yet so we stayed with Amy for three months. She put me on Dr. Fuhrman's plan. Well, it was then that my blood sugars came down from around the mid-twenties to the six or less almost consistently. This occurred in three months. Actually, it was within days that I had this noticeable difference on the Fuhrman plan. However, when we moved to our new home, I couldn't stay on it. It was just too bland for me or maybe I wasn't as committed. I went on for about three years that way.

Then, Amy started considering Dr. McDougall. It was Amy who was the push, the thrust to get us all healthy. She said, "You have got to try this." Well, we did try it and it did work. It brought my blood sugars down. I felt better. I started to lose weight. We inherited some money from an aunt and Carol said, "Let's take the whole family to Dr. McDougall's program in Santa Rosa California. We'll make it a health vacation for the family." It's a 10-day session at Dr. McDougall's program. My son Brian, my daughter Kate, my daughter Amy, my wife Carol and myself – we all attended the 10-day session. We learned how to cook. We learned how to make things interesting and tasty and attractive. As a result, when we came back from that program, I had lost 16 pounds in the 10 days. We continued the program when we got back. We were really dedicated to it because we saw the power of this for many people. For me, it was learning about the science behind everything.

Dr. McDougall had a unique way of presenting the plan, how to incorporate it into your life and supporting it with the science behind it all. He had the support of references to a lot of studies that had been done. One example that sticks in my mind is to imagine that milk from a cow is designed specifically to make a young calf gain 400 pounds in six months. That milk is not made for human consumption. If you want to gain 400 pounds in six months, continue to drink milk. It is logical. It really isn't made for us.

Then, he showed a video. This was about fat and oil. It was inside an artery and it showed someone who had just eaten oil and how the oil caused the actual cells to swell and start laying down deposits of plaque along the sides of the artery walls. Dr. McDougall said, "Just imagine you get up in the morning and you have bacon and eggs. You are laying fat down in your arteries. It takes 10 hours for the fat to dissipate or start to clear. Then you have lunch time, four hours later and you have a cheeseburger. You are laying more fat down. Then, for dinner, you have a steak or a chicken breast. They all have fat and grease in them. So, you are laying more and more fat down in your arteries. Your body never gets a chance to heal itself." That made a lot of sense to me, just seeing that video of what happens when you eat fat or grease or oil. It was seeing those things that caused me to get his books, read the books and understand how our bodies can heal themselves.

Because of McDougall's program, my diabetes started to reverse. I was on Metformin in the morning. I was also on Januvia and Glycoside. I don't take them anymore. I take only one shot of insulin now. Dr. McDougall said to me, "You are not really a type 2 diabetic. I am going to call you a type 1.5 diabetic. You are always going to need a little bit of insulin but you don't need to be on all these other drugs." The side effects to those medications are bad.

We stuck to the plan for a year. Although I hadn't had a hamburger in almost a year and a half, we were in California again. We were at the three day Advanced Study Weekend with Dr. McDougall. I tried a Carl's Junior Three-way Burger. It was one of the best burgers I have ever had, but it didn't really satisfy me. Why did I do that? It was a stupid thing to do. I guess I had to find that out. I talked to somebody from McDougall's program and they said you are going to have those days where you do go off, but, the trick is you have got to get right back on it. Knowing how well the plan works makes it so much easier for me to get back on it.

The thing about the plan is you must prepare your meals in advance. I always make a huge Instant Pot full of vegetable chili and I've always got lunch. When I start getting the urge to eat something, I've got it ready right there. I can put a big container in the fridge and I've got another one ready to go as soon as that one is empty. That is how I can stay on track. I don't need a lot of diversity in my food. I can live on baked potatoes, vegetable chili, and the occasional beer. That is my story. I had always been fat. This has given me a chance. I haven't been less than 200 pounds for most of my life. Now I am down to 171 pounds.

How much weight have you lost?

In total, I have lost 108 pounds. I feel much better, obviously. I don't get winded going up and down stairs now. I can bend over and tie my shoe laces without passing out. I feel stronger. I feel healthier. Dr. McDougall's daughter, Heather, asked me to write something for the program based on what our family had experienced. I just sent them a quick e-mail with a couple of paragraphs about how we have all felt so much better. We've been losing the weight and our bodies are responding beautifully to this very positive way of eating. We are all feeling healthier. I feel stronger now than I have in a long time even though I'm half the size I used to be.

Did you notice any changes in your clarity, any difference in your thinking?

That is hard to say because four years ago I had a TIA, a trans-ischemic attack, like a mini stroke. I was very fortunate. I have very little residual effect, other than my left hand has very little feeling in it. I have forgotten some things I should remember like people's names. Names I should have known for years but I have this dead spot in my brain. I have real trouble pulling them out sometimes. It is hard to say if my brain was affected by the food because it was affected adversely by the mini stroke. I do believe my memory would be worse if I wasn't on this plan. I haven't had any recurrences of a stroke. This is a good thing because the doctors say people who have had a TIA will, within a short period of time afterwards, experience a more serious stroke. Touch wood.

That won't happen now because your healthy diet is clearing out the plaque and sludge in the arteries going to your brain.

Exactly. That is part and parcel of why I want to stay on plan. I belong to a motorcycle riding group, and on Wednesday nights we get together in Hamilton at the Foolin' Flaggin and I'll have a Guinness. The first couple of times I had the carrot and celery and vegetable plate. Last week, I had some chicken wings... with nothing on them, but still deep fried. They came with a serving of guilt with every bite I took.

I don't want it to become a habit because we are so good. We have been perfect on the plan for one year and two months. We haven't let go of it once. When we travelled to Portugal, we found it challenging to have food with no oil, but we managed. The Portuguese were very accommodating. They would go out of their way to get us boiled potatoes or baked potatoes and steamed vegetables.

What was your family's experience at the McDougall Program?

Amy, Carol, and I were very pleased with the results. What I have discovered is exactly what Dr. McDougall has said. The fat you put in here (pointing to his mouth) is the fat that shows up here (pointing to his bottom). The benefits of not eating meat are great. I do consider the impact of meat production on our environment. The farming of animals for food is doing some drastic things. People don't understand that. That information has been suppressed, hidden under the carpet. What goes on behind closed doors in slaughterhouses is kept hush-hush. Don't tell anybody so nobody really knows.

Why is it that this plan shows such great results as opposed to the lobbyist version of the Canadian food guide? Why is that? I asked Dr. McDougall that and he said, "It is not a conspiracy, Dan. It is just about money." I said, "Well, I am a police officer. That is what constitutes a conspiracy." That is basically the way I am looking at it now. The lobbyists are poisoning us as a nation, both in the US and Canada. Probably, the rest of the world is exposed to a lobbyist version of a healthy diet and I don't know what the answer is. Dr. McDougall has battled these lobbyists for about 40 years. I am so glad to see he is still trying, but he must be deflated because the message still hasn't gotten through.

This message must get through. This should be taught to our children. They are killing themselves by eating the McDonald's version of food: the fat and the grease in there, the dairy products with the carcinogens that are in them. From what I can see, I don't think I would have been able to keep up a strong front the way Dr. McDougall has. He has dealt with a lot of adversaries and has run into all kinds of opposition to his program. They are there. They are Big Money, the meat lobby, the chicken lobby, the dairy lobby, fish lobby, the you-name-it lobby, that create our national food guides. It is criminal. Nobody is being held responsible.

Your daughter introduced you to Dr. McDougall. Out of all the reading and research that you have done, who else has inspired you?

Other than following Dr. Fuhrman's program for a short time, I really haven't looked at other people. I remember seeing the slides that Dr. McDougall used where he said, "Dr. Atkins, FAT & DEAD. Dr. So-and-so, FAT & DEAD!" All these famous diets and these physicians weren't healthy and are no longer alive. Whereas, "Dr. Fuhrman: SLIM & VEGAN, Dr. McDougall: SLIM & VEGAN, Dr. Greger: SLIM & VEGAN, Dr. Esselstyn: SLIM & VEGAN, Dr. Barnard: SLIM & VEGAN, Dr. Campbell: SLIM & VEGAN." Also, all of them are alive and thriving, and living well into old age. There is something to be said about this truth.

We went back to the McDougall's Advanced Study Weekend for the three-day event in June of this year. We listen to them. Dr. Dean Ornish was one. There was another doctor there who presented another opinion on it. He took a little bit of a beating at this conference. I went up to him afterwards and said, "I appreciate your point of view because I think we must be objective, as opposed to subjective." I have always been a believer that a person who reads one book is a very dangerous person. A person who reads many books gets a more objective assessment of things. The books that I have read on this topic support what Dr. McDougall is presenting to us. That is why I am a firm believer.

I thank my daughter Amy for steering me in this direction and making me a healthier person. I don't know if I would have had another stroke had I not been on this plan, but I think personally, I feel better. I feel stronger. That has got to count for something.

When you cook, are you following Dr. McDougall's recipes?

Occasionally, but I like to experiment. That is what I heard him say. Experiment. Try different spices and different ingredients. Every time I make a vegetable chili, I experiment a bit with the different spices. My wife Carol says that every time I do, I make it better. Now I know what combination of spices to use to make it quite tasty. I enjoy that sort of thing. I am not really a recipe follower. Maybe I don't have the patience to do it. I'm a dump a can of this in there, chop up some celery, chop up something else and throw it in there. These Instant Pots, they are fantastic. They have made cooking so easy. With the Instant Pot, we don't have to spend half a day getting a meal ready.

I think Jeff Novick, the registered dietitian at Dr. McDougall's program, was another person who inspired me. He told us to make it simple. It doesn't have to be complex. You can eat well and very healthily without spending hours in the kitchen. He said, throw some rice on. Throw some mixed vegetables in it. Spice it up a little bit with some cumin, garlic, and some celery salt, and you have a great meal. I have learned how to sauté in water, or dry sauté just with the natural moisture from the vegetables. You just have to be much more careful than slathering them with oil to keep them from burning. I enjoy cooking, even though I don't really believe I'm cooking because it's so easy. I'm simply putting ingredients together to make something that I find palatable.

What difficulties or obstacles have you faced?

One of the obstacles is I am easily swayed in stressful situations. If Carol asks me to get her some potato chips, I will go get the potato chips because I want them too. I'll acquiesce because that is my favorite snack. That is an obstacle that I'm getting over. I am learning how to say no. I have learned to think of the benefits rather than the instant gratification. The momentary satisfaction that you might get from having salt and oil doesn't compare to the health benefits of the program.

We cook with very little salt. I never have been a person that needed salt on my meal. The only time I ever put a little salt on is when I make a tomato sandwich, a little bit of salt on the tomato with lots of pepper to give it a little bit of a bite. The sandwich bread I use is always multigrain. I like those flat thin breads. I'll have one of those with a thick slice of tomato, lettuce, salt and pepper. That will satisfy me for lunch. One of the things we found we enjoy is soup with a meal, as Dr. McDougall suggests. It starts to fill you up and you don't eat as much. I have always loved potatoes. This is the perfect lifestyle plan for me because I love potatoes. I can eat potatoes until the cows come home and I don't gain weight. It is amazing. Potatoes get such a bad rap, that they're so fattening, but it's not true. I'm living proof of that. I do enjoy a beer now and then. Dr. McDougall said that is acceptable. I don't make a habit out of it. Like I said, on Wednesdays, I go out with the guys and I have a pint of Guinness, which I love and I am satisfied for the week.

Are there any friends or family members who disagree with your McDougall lifestyle?

No. We do keep in mind something Jeff Novick says, "Don't become disciples of this program. People will learn to hate you." We would mention what we were doing to our friends, but not make a big deal out of it. You can turn people off so easily.

A big obstacle is exercise. We have a hard time keeping to a schedule of activity. We'd rather just sit around and watch TV. Of course, that gets us to thinking about having a snack. Nowadays, instead of grabbing something I shouldn't be eating, I get a big glass of ice water and fill myself up with that. The last few nights I had eight to ten glasses of water in the evening watching TV. That also wakes me up in the middle of the night a few times too, but at least I didn't eat the potato chips!

What about your doctor?

After I had the TIA, I was recommended to another specialist here in town. When I told him about the Dr. McDougall plan he said, "That guy is a quack. He is a snake oil salesman." I didn't say it to him, but I wanted to say it. I am thinking to myself, "I am looking around your waiting room here. All of your patients are obese and on walkers and in wheel chairs, and what are you doing for them?" I feel great, thanks to my quack, snake oil doctor. All this specialist guy is, is a pill pusher. I went back to my doctor and told him I don't want to go to this doctor anymore. I felt like a lab rat. He tried so many medicines on me that didn't work. One of them almost killed me because I had such an adverse reaction to it. I thought to myself, I don't need this guy. He is experimenting on me.

I have gone back to my family physician. He insists that I be strict about taking my blood glucose levels regularly. Dr. McDougall said, "You don't die of high blood sugar. You die of low blood sugars. As long as you keep it under 8, you should be okay. Don't check it throughout the day. All that does is cause you to become anxious, and it may cause you to not eat properly and go down into hypoglycemia." That is when you go too low, and that is when people die.

I am living the Dr. McDougall plan. I feel great, my vision hasn't suffered. I go regularly to the optometrist, and she says there is no damage because of the diabetes. I am fortunate there. There isn't any damage to my kidneys, which very often accompanies diabetes. I am good there. I think Dr. McDougall's recommendations are much more reasonable than the extreme ideas of a lot of other physicians who are peddling pills. I am not taking any of those drugs anymore, so there are no side effects. My diabetes is at a standstill, steady as she goes. I am not on a downward spiral like most people with diabetes.

My weight is the lowest it's ever been since I was a kid. Plus, it wasn't a struggle to lose it either. It was easy. It fell off. It was a sideline to getting healthy with this program. There is no struggle to maintain it either. I can eat as many potatoes as I want and still lose weight. That is one of the good things that I like. I have learned how to cook foods that I used to not like. Now, I can make them flavorful and I enjoy them. It is funny how your taste buds become more acute to the natural flavors of the food. I probably didn't eat beans prior to this program. Now, I love all kinds of beans. I cook with every kind of bean imaginable. I love the flavors.

When you told your family doctor you were going to follow the McDougall program, what did he say?

I didn't tell him that I was going to Dr. McDougall's Live-In Program. I told him when I came back. He was happy that I had lost weight and that my sugars were down. He said, "Keep doing what you are doing. It's working."

Who took you off your medication?

I did. McDougall suggested that I go off them. I said, "The doctor in the states has told me I should be off of these medications and I no longer want them." The specialist I was going to see in town said, "I don't advise that." I said, "I don't want to take them anymore." He said, "Okay, but I am not advising you to go off of them." I talked to my doctor here and he said, "It's working for you. Your blood sugars are down. You are feeling healthy. You are losing the weight. Keep doing what works." That is why I like my physician. He is a little more open minded. I think a lot of physicians get trapped in a paradigm and they are not willing to see what is happening in the rest of the world. I call it tunnel vision. They don't want to look at what else is possible. It is what they were taught.

My son, Brian, has gone through medical school. He was a nutritionist before he went into medicine. He said he was so glad he was a nutritionist because in medical school you get a six-hour lecture on nutrition and that is it. That is what most doctors get. They know nothing about nutrition.

Dr. Greger would say he's got a great tool of nutrition in his medical tool kit. Brian went with you to see Dr. McDougall. That must have been phenomenal for him.

It was. He didn't have the same dedication to it but then he was already very fit. He has always had healthy big muscles and bone structure. He is a big, healthy-looking man. I don't know where he got it from, maybe my dad. My dad was a big man, too. I took after my mother, a little shorter in stature and a little stouter. Brian understands the role nutrition plays in our health, and he believes nutrition can be more of a preventative thing than treating the symptoms with pills.

Where is your support coming from?

My support is coming primarily from my family - mostly Carol and my two daughters. My son is so busy with his medical practice. I don't see him very often. When we go out for dinner as a family, we are not going to have a steak or a chicken breast. We are going to have some vegetables, and a baked potato, and maybe some rice pasta. We do go to Thai restaurants a lot because they offer what we want. We can say to the chef we don't want any oil, and they are very accommodating in most restaurants. We often phone ahead to restaurants to make sure we can get the kind of meal we want without the oil.

Do you have any advice for beginners?

You have to be persistent. In other words, don't expect things to happen overnight. It takes nine minutes to do a perfect large potato in the microwave. If you want it crispy on the outside, you throw it in the oven for another ten minutes, and it crisps up and you have a wonderful meal.

For a summer barbecue or a wedding, we'll prepare ahead and take our food with us. When we go to a dinner party, we'll say don't prepare anything for us. We'll bring our own food. It has come to the point where some other friends of ours are experimenting. They are starting to enjoy the sort of food we like because they have enjoyed the food that we brought. We make enough for everybody. If they want to try it, great, if not, we bring it back home and have leftovers. Don't throw it out. We are going to a wedding next month, and we will bring our meal with us.

With this kind of lifestyle, have you thought about animal rights and the environment?

Before McDougall, I had no idea how animal agriculture is impacting the environment. I've watched several films like, *Vegucated* and *Forks over Knives*, that talk about the negative impact of animal agriculture on our planet. We must be looking at this as a global population. It is frustrating because Big Money is behind animal agriculture practices and it is hard to fight Big Money. What can I do as an individual? Well, I can stay on the plan. Just one day at a time. We do what we can do. Also, the only other thing we can do is try to convince people without being overly zealous, that a whole food plant-based diet is the route to go.

I have to admit I have never really thought about animal rights. I have grown up in a society where animals were basically propagated to be a food source. I hate seeing some of the conditions that animals are raised in for food. They are deplorable in many cases. Some are more humane than others but I have realized we don't need to eat animals to survive on this planet.

What we are doing is like the automobile industry. They are building automobiles and stock piling them in fields. They are not even being sold. They won't sell them. It is for the jobs to keep people employed and a lot of this meat production is the same. All the meat doesn't get eaten. All the chicken doesn't get eaten. Where does it go? It goes into dump sites, but it keeps people employed. That seems to be the big thrust in this world. We have got to keep people employed even if it harms our environment. It is not something that is right there in front of you all the time.

Those poor animals are suffering and the only way I can help them is to not eat them. That in turn does not support the system.

Encouraging other people to consider this way of eating, as well as me and my family continuing to follow a plant-based diet will be one way to help the animals.

My one grandson decided on his own volition to become a vegetarian because he didn't want to see the animals get hurt. He has been a vegetarian since the age of four. A lot of kids are that way and isn't it wonderful that he is in a home where his point of view is respected. He has freedom of choice.

Do you see yourself changing the world in any other way?

I think by eating this diet, I'm helping to change the world. That is the biggest thing I think we can do. I am not going to be a crusader like Dr. McDougall. I don't have the background to do that. All I can say is, it works for me. It works for my wife. It works for my daughter. We are an example of the fact that you can lose weight even though you have tried every other diet plan on the planet and it hasn't worked. This is not a diet plan, it is a health plan with a side effect of losing weight. Plus, the weight stays off if you stay on the plan. When have you ever been on any other plan where you didn't have to work to keep the weight from coming back? I have been steadily losing weight. I haven't quite reached my goal weight yet. I still have ten more pounds to go. I would like to get down another ten pounds to where I was at my lowest weight. That's the weight where I felt my best.

Did you have to switch to McDougall's Program for Maximum Weight Loss to lose weight?

No, I just do *The Starch Solution*. It may seem unfair to those who must take a strict approach, but for me the weight just naturally comes off and I feel really good.

What are your future plans related to the McDougall Program?

My plan is to continue with this program for the rest of my life. I also expect to ride into Sturgis, South Dakota, on a motorcycle at 95 years of age. That is my plan.

Do you have anything else to add?

I am so impressed with all the dietitians, doctors, nutritionists, and even a PhD from a university, who presented at the Live-In Program and Advanced Study Weekend that we went to. There are so many phenomenal healthcare professionals who are supporting this lifestyle with science. The wave is coming. We are at the cutting edge of this whole movement. The world is beginning to embrace a plant-eating lifestyle. More and more people are talking about it. The news, talk programs, people are actually talking about whole food plant-based diets. It is catching on.

My final thought is that in my family, we all lost weight on the McDougall plan, and losing weight was a big part of it. Even though that is not the prime objective, it was one of the objectives that made the program attractive to us. We are getting slim and we are getting healthy and strong. We can eat the foods we love. Best of all, we are never hungry.

Chapter Twelve
Cecilia

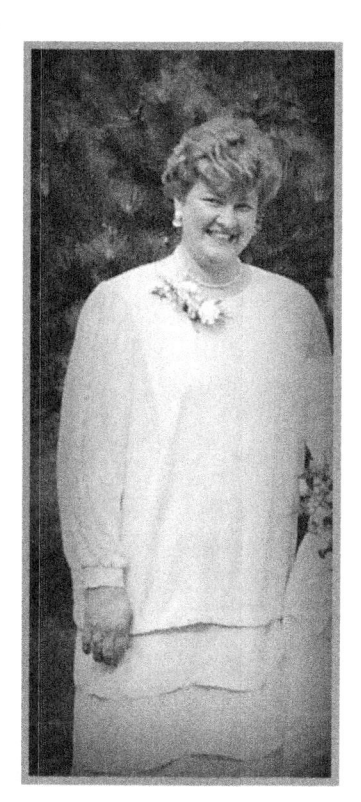

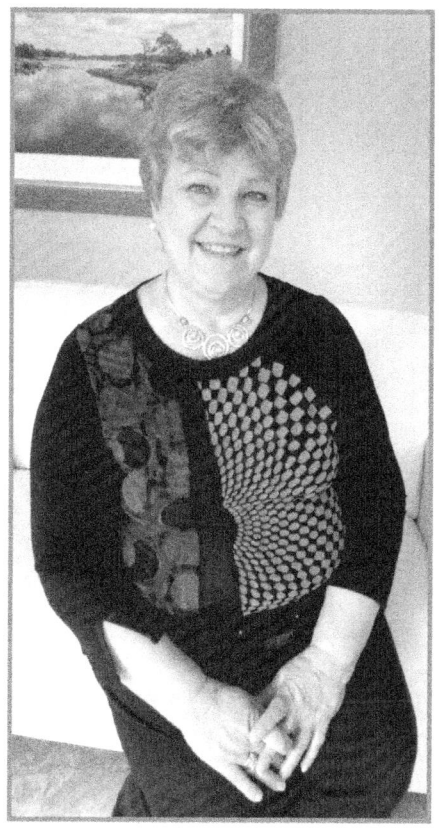

Cecilia's brother discovered Dr. McDougall while searching for a diet to help with his own arthritis, and recommended it to his sister. She decided to give it a try. After attending a three-day McDougall workshop in California, she discovered how easy it is to lose weight on the program, and clear up the osteoarthritis in her knees.

Chapter Twelve - Cecilia's Interview

Can you tell us, Cecilia, a little bit about your personal background and what you do?

I am the CEO of a production company which manufacture flags. Our flag company is 51 years old and my parents started it. I am the president and I have 14 employees. I work between three locations. This is our 20th year, that I have been president. I am divorced now. I have two sons, one is 30 and one is 29. My ex-husband is Irish. We have lots of starch in our world. Now, for the last nine years, I have been going out with an Italian man. He and I live separately, but we do share a house together in Italy. We go to Italy for a few months of the year. Irish and Italian foods are mostly my life.

Well, as they say, "You don't inherit diseases, you inherit diets." Can you tell us how you found Dr. McDougall and how you started with his program?

It was because of my younger brother that I learned about Dr. McDougall. I am the eldest of eight kids. My brother has juvenile arthritis and he's suffered his whole life with this terrible affliction. I am 60, he is 55. He and his wife are always looking into alternative therapies. They have been married for 35 years. She is convinced that his recovery is all about diet. He doesn't take any pills, but he is totally crippled with arthritis. She wanted him to try a different diet because none of this other stuff has been working. He came across Dr. McDougall himself. He is a world traveller and lives in the Middle East.

Fed Up with Being Fat and Sick

He said, "I am going to go to California and find out what this whole McDougall thing is all about." He went there for the 10-day program, and came back totally inspired.

While he was there, he met a woman named Yvonne, who was about 27 years old at the time. She weighed close to 400 pounds. He befriended her because she looked like my niece. They sat beside each other for meals and things. Ed got a lot out of the 10-day workshop. That was very intense.

Then what happened, a year and a half after he went the workshop, he got an email from this girl Yvonne, saying, "Hey, I am just cleaning out my computer and I see a picture of the two of us standing beside Dr. McDougall. That was then and this is me now." She forwarded a picture of herself. She had lost 170 pounds. She said she had left the workshop and she was determined to stay on the plan. She decided she was going to change her life around. I would never have believed it if I hadn't seen the pictures of Yvonne for myself. My brother had sent me the pictures and said, "Cecelia, this McDougall Program thing really works and if you are thinking about losing weight, look at this girl, Yvonne. Here she is in her exercise outfit. She is doing yoga and she is just a very happy woman." That encouraged me to look into Dr. McDougall's program. I realized there is something there for me, so I got on a plane and went to California. I went on a three-day workshop with Dr. McDougall.

When did you go?

I went in May of 2016. The food was totally prepared and the event took place at a wonderful hotel. The famous actress, Jean Harlow, used to stay at this hotel. It was an old-fashioned hotel with the beautiful swimming pool in the middle, and a restaurant attached to it that we didn't use. We had all our food brought in and prepared in their hotel kitchens. Everything was taken care of, from snacks to intense workshops. Breakfast was served at 7:30, the lectures started at 9 a.m. and it didn't stop until 10 o'clock at night. So, I learned a lot of things. I brought chocolate bars, chips, and a lot of things in my suitcase with me, thinking I am not going to be able to possibly manage McDougall's food, but I did manage. I enjoyed the food and it totally satisfied my hunger. Plus, I had no cravings.

My biggest thing is chicken. I miss chicken, but they showed me tofu. I had never tried tofu before. And gravy, here was this big pitcher of gravy you can have with mashed potatoes. I was really inspired by that.

Who were the speakers that inspired you?

Oh, I can't member the names of the speakers. Almost everybody had worked with Dr. McDougall over the years. One was a marketing guy, which was something I am interested in. A few were doctors, and a couple of nurses. Mary, his wife, gave a couple of talks. Dr. McDougall was great, but Mary was practical. That's what I needed to hear. What happens when I go to Costco? I go to Costco for everybody else: my family, my mother, my kids, everybody else, so I asked her, "Do I just walk past all this food?" She said, "I just love going to Costco too. I love going out for breakfasts. I love having Mexican food." Everything she said was inspiring to me. She said "Get this and get that, and get this. This is okay on this diet, as a side dish." I walked out of there totally inspired and didn't look back.

I left Dr. McDougall's workshop and I went to Las Vegas. I went to Vegas by myself thinking, "Oh I'm just going to be here for a day and a half." I was so inspired by Dr. McDougall that I didn't go into any of the buffets or anything else that I would usually do. I said, "This is it. I am doing this diet right away, right now." I came back home after my day and a half in Vegas and jumped right into *The Starch Solution*. I was just eating potatoes and rice in Vegas. I was very proud of myself for that day and a half, sticking to the program despite the holiday location.

When I came back to Barrie and to my mother, who at the time, had been living with me for 22 years, I said, "Mom, I am sorry, I know you need your protein and I know you need your cheese, your milk, your chicken and everything every day. I have to prepare this for you, but I am not following that diet anymore. I am going to stick with Dr. McDougall's Program." She was a real trooper. She said, "Okay Cecelia, I will do the same."

Well, unfortunately she didn't think that way for very long. She soon wanted chicken every day and she started calling my sister across the road, saying, "Cecelia's not giving me chicken." My sister would bring over chicken and cheese or whatever for my mother. She did slip back to her old ways after about three weeks. That was okay. She was very encouraging for me.

My Irish father, since I was a kid growing up, insisted on having a pot of potatoes on the stove every day. I am battling celiac disease. With the celiac side of things, I was always constantly making sure there was no gluten in anything, and potatoes are gluten-free so that is a good thing. I did McDougall's Starch Solution program up until the beginning of August. I lost 17 pounds, from May 10th until August 8th. I lost those 17 pounds. Every day I was jumping for joy as I jumped on that scale.

Have you ever experienced anything like that in your life before this program? I remember doing weight loss programs where I would drag myself up to the scale and peel off all the layers, hoping it will make a difference.

I always yell at my scale too. I step on it and yell, "liar, liar, liar!" This time it felt so good. I was so excited because you always knew the numbers were going down with such little effort, and not feeling hungry all the time.

Was your primary goal for going to see Dr. McDougall to lose weight and make sure you didn't have any other health issues?

I had sore knees, and so I went to the hospital and I said, "My knee really hurts. I think I banged it." He took an x-ray and said, "Oh no, it is osteoarthritis." I said, "When is that going to happen?" He said, "You have it now." I was so surprised.

I just turned 60 in June, a month after I did the workshop. The sore knees went away almost immediately when I started the McDougall diet. That has stayed away. This way of eating has been a great relief to my joints.

What happened next? We are at August 8th.

Yes, I had gone to Rome, Italy, and my boyfriend, who is a wonderful man and the best cook in the world, in my opinion, was so happy for me doing the diet. However, he believes like most Italians that you should have a teaspoon of olive oil every morning when you wake up, just to keep your bones limber. Italians don't believe in butter. That was one of the hardest things to give up, butter, on the McDougall program. I love butter.

The thing is, when I wasn't looking, my boyfriend would sneak olive oil on everything and anything. "Don't tell me you can't have olive oil. You have to have olive oil." So we would make gluten-free pasta, which he was always great about eating. But when I wasn't looking, he was putting a teaspoon or two of olive oil on top of the pasta. He also uses an awful lot of salt, like two teaspoons of salt, to season the pasta. I just finally gave up because everything was just too tempting.

Our town in Italy is a meat town. Everything centers around sheep and goat. In Italy, every day they must have meat, and the butcher was right across the road from us. My boyfriend would bring home six pork chops or whatever it was, you know, like prosciutto. I eventually just gave up trying to fight it. I thought, "I'll just wait until I get back to Canada, and start up again when I'm back home."

I was so glad to get the connection with you, because I needed that. It is inspiring to be with everybody who is doing this McDougall lifestyle.

Are there any other people besides Dr. McDougall that have been inspiring you? Like Jeff Novick?

Jeff was there. He was a very good speaker. He was inspiring. He brought humor into his presentations, which was great. There were a couple of dry speakers that were showing graphs and stuff.

I am terrible at that stuff. There were a lot of people from the 10-day workshop who had returned for the three-day just to top up. There were wives there who had brought their husbands along. "Come on, let's make a little holiday of this." Somebody drove all the way from Florida, in their motor home, to California. There were lots of people from California. Maybe they were there for the third or fourth time, just to meet people.

The food was fantastic, just fantastic. Being of Irish decent I love to eat oatmeal every day. Mary was telling us that she buys *Uncle Bob's Oatmeal* steal cut oats from Costco. I went out to Costco and bought a big bag of that, and I cook it in my rice cooker. I cook that, as soon as I get to work and that lasts me for two days. She said that fruit and oatmeal is their breakfast too. I love the nut milks. I am lactose-free. It was easy for me to switch over to soy milk.

Do you ever go on YouTube and watch the lectures of these doctors who are leading the way in plant-based nutrition, like Dr. Michael Greger, Dr. Neal Barnard, or Dr. T. Colin Campbell?

At this point, I have only watched Dr. McDougall. Yvonne, the woman that has lost all of this weight sent me a note saying, "This was really hard for me because I am young. When I would go out with my girlfriends partying I knew it was going to be difficult. So, this is what I did, for the first few months, I only ate potatoes. I couldn't believe how that was sustainable for me. I could get along just fine, eating mashed potatoes. I didn't have time to cook, and then I went online to watch the different videos on YouTube about cooking."

Dr. McDougall has *The Starch Solution* program and then he has a stricter version that is called, *The McDougall Program for Maximum Weight Loss*.

Yes, that was the one Yvonne was talking about.

The difference is *The McDougall Program for Maximum Weight Loss* is designed to help you lose weight quickly and efficiently.

I found it difficult to drink a lot of water. I found it difficult to give up coffee. Of course, I have cream in my coffee. Dr. McDougall said to us, as soon as we got there, "I know there is a Starbucks right across the road and you all want your caffeine. I think that it is poison, but if you want to go get some, just don't have any cream. Have a light coffee, and make sure it is coffee, not decaffeinated coffee. The chemicals they add to take the caffeine out will kill you." We would all run over there and get our small coffee, and he was standing there shaking his head going no, no, no. Mary, who was standing right behind him, was motioning, "Oh go on, go ahead." He did say that he understood the changes were difficult, especially in the beginning, and Mary's in the background signalling, "Go on."

Have you seen *Mary's Mini* on YouTube? You just eat one starch, morning, noon and night with no fruit and no vegetables. You pick porridge, or you pick potatoes, or you pick rice and that is all you eat. It is all about simplicity. Just like your dad, putting

on a pot of potatoes on the stove. That is all you need to eat. It is what you can survive on. All the vitamins are there.

My father was eating them like a round snowball. He'd eat a round potato cold like that. You can survive on it if you want to, but I would imagine you'd get bored with it eventually.

Where are you today? Are you 50 percent starch-based?

Oh yes, I'd say I am about 65 percent starch-based right now. Gluten is not part of my world, having to be gluten-free. This diet is a good companion for celiac disease. That is why my brother really encouraged me. "You have enough challenges already. Try this Dr. McDougall plan because it is made for celiacs. You love the rice and potatoes and corn products like polenta." I love polenta. My brother said, *"The Starch Solution* program is made for you." The only meat I will eat is chicken, and that's only when I go out. I'll admit, that is going to be a hard thing to give up, once I start again. I just boiled up six eggs a week ago. That is going to be hard for me to give up, too. I know that I can get into it. I know the success. That success is just astounding!

I have never really tried to lose weight before. I have always been a big girl. I am 5 foot 10 and I have always been overweight, but I feel very healthy. It has never been a real need. I never felt so fat that I wanted to lose weight. But I know I have to, because my father died at the age of 53 from a massive heart attack and he was a big man, 6 foot 3, and he was overweight. When he was young, he was a figure skater and he was a bike rider and he was active all the time. The rest of my siblings are all thin except one and she said, "Figure out how to lose the weight and tell me what I have to do. Cook for me and bring it in to work for me and I'll eat it!"

During the three-day workshop, I left one lecture because it was dry and I was bored. I bumped into Dr. McDougall outside the dining room. He invited me to join him for lunch. It was amazing. We spent an entire hour together. He said something very interesting. He said, "The bottom line is, just eat starch. Don't make it more difficult than it really is." I forget that and I think, I've got to add this and do that, add the right kind of flour, etc., but like he said, just make it simple. Just eat starch.

What is it going to take for you personally to get back on the program 100 percent? What are your obstacles? Is it a matter of waking up one morning and deciding I am doing this?

That is how I am going to do it. Like when I came back from the three days in California, I decided that this is the way it is. It will happen again. I had no idea what the impact of the Italian food was going to have on me. I had no idea I was going to get so much resistance from my boyfriend. I can't cook Italian, so he has to cook it. He sneaks things into the food or else we are sitting there and he says, "I have to have my meat. I am sorry."

The biggest challenge for many people seems to be with the people who are not supporting them. Many people are in the same boat as you.

That is why it was so nice to be at this workshop because everybody was struggling with similar things. They brought their partner, so their partners could start seeing the results of others. They came to see if it was something they'd be willing to try. There must have been 200 people in the workshop, and many of them were couples. Typically, there would be one person who was there for themselves and they were trying to encourage their partner to change as well. There were also a lot of mother-daughter teams.

Have you got a January plan? Have you got plans to start the *Starch Solution* program again?

I am off to Italy again. I love going to Italy. My boyfriend is part of a big festive team celebration so he is going back there four times this year. I am only going in January and July this year. The day I come back is the day I am starting. That is it! This is exciting. It is easy. I know what to do.

There is another problem with living in Italy, it's the coffee. We live next door to a coffee bar. We spend three to four hours a day there, and the espresso is hard to resist.

But if that was the only thing that you did, having the espresso, how is that going to impede your weight loss?

Dr. McDougall says coffee bars should be called poison bars. You are just drinking poison. He was adamant that you should not be drinking coffee. I felt this was going to be a huge hurdle for me. I don't know if I am ready to give up coffee.

What things on the program do you like to eat?

Well, rice is my favorite. The white and the brown, I am mixing the two of them together now. I love pepper, white or red. I love pepper and rice. Then I will throw vegetables in it, like broccoli. It all goes in the rice cooker first thing in the morning. I'll scoop away at that all day long. That is my absolute favorite and it is also easy on my stomach. I don't put any sauce on it.

I like mashed potatoes. I make Mary's gravy with mashed potatoes. It is so delicious. When I am on the program, I make a great big container of the gravy and then I freeze small portions of it in the ice tray. As I needed it, I would thaw out a gravy cube and have little bits of gravy now and again.

Rice cakes and peanut butter are a favorite, but you shouldn't have too much peanut butter. I have porridge for breakfast every day with fruit like blueberries. I love the sparkling water. I have never been a pop drinker but if I ever felt like I needed to have something sweet, I would get sparkling water with lime or lemon in it. I would drink that maybe three times a week. I am not a recipe follower. I make things very simple and this is not hard to follow. That is my base.

When you start again, how are you going to handle your boyfriend? Do you see him during the week?

We only spend weekends together. I can follow the plan during the week and then on the weekends, if I goof up, it is not as serious. He does have to have pasta every single day so we will have pasta every day we're together on Fridays, Saturdays and Sundays. He can keep his sauce off to the side, and I'll have it white (without sauce), with salt and pepper on it. I'll chop in tomatoes and all of that. He just hates to see me contaminate a perfectly proper Italian recipe. He always wants to know what I am going to put in the pasta, and he thinks those vegetables will ruin it.

Is there a way you can enrol him to support you, by explaining to

him the health benefits?

I have tried everything. He is very stubborn. His English is fantastic, but when he doesn't want to hear it, he starts reverting into Italian. It is absolutely adorable. He is a big man. He's tall, and he's a big eater. He is supportive in many things. We both have our own businesses. We support each other in business. He did love to see that I lost some weight. He never said to me, "You are too big." He did compliment me when I lost the 17 pounds. "My goodness, look at you." That was lovely. I think he will come around to it eventually, especially if I stick to it, and he gets used to it.

Did you have any issues with co-workers when you were following this program last summer?

Yes, good issues. I have three co-workers. One followed it right away and then went away for the summer. She said that if I go back on, she'll go back on. I have somebody at work to go along with me. And my niece at work, she said, "We'll see how the others do." Once she sees results, she will do the same thing.

As for my other co-workers, they are fantastic. I have my own shelf in the fridge because of my celiac side of things. They have always been aware of my diet restrictions, and this is just another part of it. I am getting lots of support at work.

When I went to Italy, I told my mom she had to go on respite care, because she can't be at home by herself. There is just the two of us in this big house. So, she went into a retirement home and she loves it there and wants to stay. I miss her like crazy. As soon as I got back from Italy, I called her six times a day. I was visiting her morning, noon, and night, that kind of thing. She definitely has her diet, and her restaurant food, and that is not a concern of mine anymore. No more rushing home to make her chicken. There is no more cheese in the house.

Who are you getting your support from?

Most of my support is from my friend, Dominica. Although she is doing another type of routine and diet, she is very supportive of whatever works. We have been friends since we were three years old.

Except for my boyfriend, I am not getting any resistance from other people around me. It is also convenient that I am living on my own, which makes it easier to follow the McDougall plan. One of my sons lives in London, England and the other lives in Calgary. It would be different if I had to cook for them.

Did you tell your doctor that you were going to follow the McDougall plan?

No, I didn't. I haven't seen my doctor. Well, I went and saw him last week for the first time since 2012. I feel very healthy. He was surprised that I came to see him. I had my thyroid taken out a long time ago, and I needed a referral. I had been having gum problems. I did mention to him that I was doing the McDougall plan, and he said that this diet may cause me to start getting white spots on my gums. He thought I'd have to stop the diet at that point. But so far, I've had no problems with the *Starch Solution* program.

When you are on the program, how do you problem solve weddings, restaurants and that sort of thing?

That was difficult. I found it hard to avoid the oil that is put in everything, especially the salads. I would pick away at it. Nobody ever makes hot mashed potatoes or hot rice in the summertime. It is always cold and it usually has cheese in it. So that was hard.

What did I do? I went to the Teriyaki Experience Restaurant and would have their tofu, rice, and vegetables. It was good with their bamboo shoots and broccoli. Whenever I felt the need to have a meal out, that is where I would go. I can't have the soy sauce because there is gluten in it as well as the salt. I always put a little bit of salt and pepper on things and it tastes great.

Do you pack your own food when you go over for dinner at friends or go to a party?

I do. I do the same thing when I'm travelling. I bring a suitcase full of rice cakes, gluten-free crackers, and that sort of thing. I am used to bringing my own food and I always have something with me to eat.

Do you have any advice for beginners?

Well, just take five or six starch-based items and eat them like crazy until you are sick of them. Then, do something else. Do some research. For me, the first couple of weeks, that was easy. You see the results so fast. It was fun. Just make it simple and eat lots of starches when you are hungry. I even get up in the middle of the night if I am hungry, and I eat a starch. Before, I would never eat in the middle of the night. Now, if I am hungry, I eat. Even rice cakes come to bed with me. Porridge tastes so good. I like *Uncle Bob's* steal cut oats. Everything *Uncle Bob* does is gluten-free.

What can you do now that you couldn't do before you started the program?

Walking. We don't have a car in Italy so I must walk everywhere. I walk down to the stores, walk to the market, and walk up past the funeral home. I am doing a lot more walking and not sedentary like I was before. I am also singing a lot better because of my diaphragm. I love to sing. I have more lung capacity and my diaphragm is stronger. Those are big things. When I am in the car I am singing all the time. Planning is important. If I'm out and worried that I could get hungry, I make sure to bring food with me. I am very lucky that I am not a fast-food person and I don't go to those places.

Have you noticed an impact on your mood and attitude towards life?

I used to be a very poor sleeper. Once I started losing the weight, I started sleeping better at longer stretches of time. That is a big change. You feel better when you get better sleep. I was probably in bed for seven to eight hours, but I was only sleeping two to three hours, and then waking up. I was thinking of things and writing them down, or I'd be turning on CNN. That's how I'd spend my nights. Overall, while doing the plan, I'm exercising more, walking more, and sleeping better.

What are your future goals around the McDougall Program?

When I get back from Italy, I intend to stick with it. By then, I'll have six months before I go back to Italy again. I want to lose 70 pounds more. I have not been that thin since I was in my thirties. I would also like to go back and do another three-day program with Dr. McDougall and see the people, and get inspired. My brother and I have talked about it. He wants to go back too, so we will probably go together. It is a beautiful, beautiful place in California.

Chapter Thirteen
Sabina

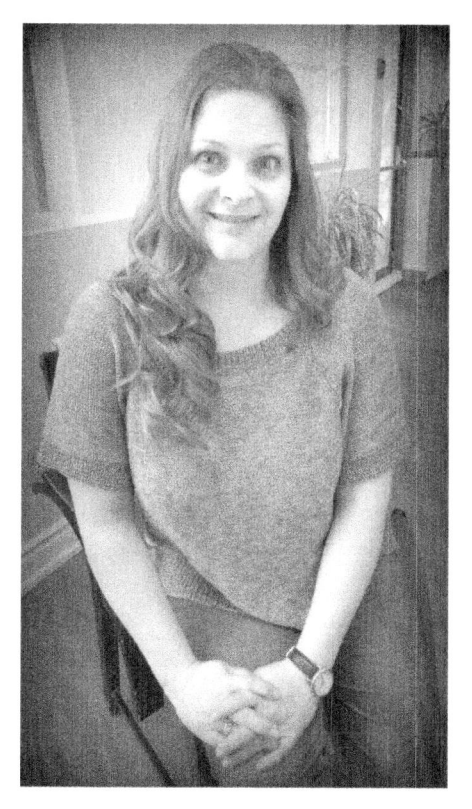

Sabina was suffering from inflammation issues and was having severe numbness and soreness on the entire right side of her body. Within days of following Dr. McDougall's program, all of Sabina's pain and inflammation vanished. In the following chapter, she discusses her greatest obstacles and success for maintaining a whole food, plant-based lifestyle.

Chapter Thirteen - Sabina's Interview

Please tell us your story, relative to Dr. McDougall's program, *The Starch Solution*.

I came to *The Starch Solution* a few years ago. I was having some inflammation issues. I had gone to the doctor for a quick visit, blood work, etc., and then I had booked a physical exam. I was having a hard time with the entire right side of my body. There was numbness and soreness, and I wasn't sleeping well. I was diagnosed with carpal tunnel in my right wrist. Basically, I was feeling miserable. I'd heard of Dr. McDougall, Dr. Barnard, and Dr. Greger. I just wanted a diet that was laid out very simply and that I could easily follow. Having been familiar with Dr. McDougall, I said I'm going to go and get one of his books – *12 Days to Dynamic Health*. It was one of his early books. I drove all the way out to Yorkdale Mall to get it, because there was only one copy left in the city. I read through it in literally one afternoon, and I committed to starting the diet right then and there. Everything was laid out perfectly. The book said within 12 days, you should feel better. Whatever is ailing you should improve or go away. Well for me, within three to four days all of my pain and issues just vanished. Going in for my physical about a month later, I had absolutely zero problems – no high cholesterol, everything was in the normal range. My doctor was saying, "Great! This issue has been resolved. Come back in three years." She was very happy with all my test results.

Have your health issues been completely resolved or are they still

resolving?

I would say they're still resolving. I still have some issues. I have noticed that even though I eat 100 percent plant-based, when I've had some oil, my issues come back. I get sore, lethargic, and I start to get pains all on the right side of my body, particularly in my arm and in my leg. But the moment I clean up my diet by taking out the oil and avoiding alcohol, within a couple of days, things are resolved. It's a great alarm for myself. I know I need to do better when I'm starting to have some inflammation and pain. It's said that all disease comes from some sort of inflammation in the body, so I try to eat as low inflammation as I can.

How did you discover Dr. McDougall's work?

I came across his website, and I thought it was great and interesting. Here's a doctor who is treating people through plant-based diets, which I thought was great. I was a huge advocate of Dr. Neal Barnard's, and Drs. Caldwell Esselstyn and T. Colin Campbell. I had read *The China Study*, but when I saw the film *Forks over Knives*, I would say that's when I looked more into Dr. McDougall. All those great heroes of mine were all in one place together. I couldn't believe it. I'd read almost everything that these doctors had put out about the science behind a plant-based diet. So, to have them all in one platform was just the most amazing thing. And, there was Dr. McDougall. He had a really great story, and an interesting take on it. The wonderful thing that I do love about Dr. McDougall is that he promotes starch, which is really the type of food that is going to fill us up. It's the fuel that our bodies use. But we've been so conditioned to stay away from carbs. "Oh, that stuff will 'kill' you." Well, yeah, you're absolutely right, it will, but that's if you're talking about pastries and things. Potatoes have carried forward so many cultures in the world. That's where your satiation comes in. Stop worrying about the potato, don't put the oil and butter on it. It's the fat which is really the problem, and not the starch itself.

You mentioned Drs. Barnard, Esselstyn and Campbell. Along with those doctors, who else has inspired you?

Dr. Michael Greger, who founded nutritionfacts.org, a really brilliant website on the science behind plant-based eating, is a big inspiration. Another fantastic person from whom I've learned a lot is Colleen

Patrick Goudreau. She talks a little about health, but she's more about fitting this into your life and not causing harm. She talks a lot about dealing with social situations. Dr. Richard Oppenlander is another big inspiration for me. Lindsay Nixon, The Happy Herbivore, is amazing. Matt Frasier, the No Meat Athlete, is really great too. There are so many people out there doing what I consider to be God's work, really, just looking out for people and for humanity. There are a number of amazing people who I consider to be mentors, whether I've met them or not. I really value the things that they have to say and the work that they're doing.

Have you been on a lengthy journey with this way of eating?

I've been vegan for eight years, and was eating a plant-based diet for some time before discovering Dr. McDougall. Once I had dropped all animal products, I started to feel amazing. I realized I had health issues that I hadn't considered to be issues, but suddenly, things miraculously went away. My digestion issues disappeared, which was fantastic. I had a lot of menstrual issues that just vanished. I couldn't believe it. I didn't need any type of medication to get me through.

Since starting *The Starch Solution* I can count on one hand the number of times I've had to take pain medication – and I don't think it's five! I broke one of my vertebrae when I was young and had back issues since. I used to joke that I was stoned for most of my childhood because I was always on some kind of drug for back pain. It was quite serious. The fact that I could get off everything is amazing. I've never been comfortable taking pills. Not having to take any pain medication is amazing. I think, by following this lifestyle, I've avoided issues that hit a lot of people as they age. I don't really like to think of it as a diet, it's more about what I eat. I've used Dr. McDougall's plan as a guideline, more than anything.

Yes, a plan usually implies that it's for a temporary period.

That's right. People often say they want to go on a diet, but they're in the wrong head space. It's about shifting from a short-term diet to a long-term lifestyle. Another one of my mentors, who goes by the name High Carb Hannah, is a favorite of mine. There's nothing polished. She has made a number of YouTube videos sharing how she came to *The Starch Solution*. She'll recommend trying one thing at a time, maybe a tweak. Know you're not going to get there overnight. Add foods that you wouldn't normally eat. The more you add plant-based foods, the less you'll eat of the animal foods and junk foods. As long as you're constantly improving and trying something new, it's only going to put you on the right path.

What difficulties or obstacles have you faced?

The biggest thing is the social aspect, particularly in my career. I work in beverage alcohol, so that means a lot of dinners out with people at restaurants which are rarely vegan-friendly. I must navigate through that challenge. I do some international travel for my work, and there's a lot of social stigma around the word "vegan". There's always someone who has something to say and they're going to teach you the error of your ways. I don't want to hear it. Just like they don't want to hear my vegan message either, which is fine. It's trying to find common ground and having people realize that you're just a person too. I love to ask, "How is what I decide to eat, what I put in my mouth, how is that affecting your life?" The answer is that it's not. Then, let's just move on and talk about something else.

How have you dealt with family and co-workers?

For the most part my family and co-workers are supportive. They may not agree with it, they may have a little fun with me but they understand this is how I've chosen to live my life. It's just something that's been accepted and is understood. My bosses are great. When we must go out, they will talk to the chefs, and we have relationships with most of these places anyway. Some of them get really excited about the challenge. They have a few things ready and when you come to the restaurant, they want to talk to you. They have a vision and want to try something, which is great. You have other chefs who may come out and be a little nervous about it, but usually once we have a conversation they realize, "Oh, that's not a big deal. Of course, I can do that! I'm a master chef!"

With my family, I've always been the odd one out, but I've always been someone who doesn't necessarily go with the mainstream. There was never any big to-do with my family, which is great. With my immediate family, they're supportive but they don't want to be a part of it. As much as I can talk to them until I'm blue in the face, I'm not going to be converting anybody. But they're more than happy to eat the yummy goodies that come out of my kitchen.

How are your parents with eating vegan at meals? Do they make vegan food for you?

My mother will try. Like me, she loves to cook, and she embraces the new culinary challenge. When she sees things in a magazine that looks delicious and is vegan, or something that she can veganize, we will make it together when I come for a visit. My father is fine with me being vegan. However, he doesn't want anything to do with veganism. If my mother's away and it's just me and him, well, he doesn't cook. If he wants to eat, he's going to eat what's being served. I'm a decent cook, and he's always loved what I've served for him. I have a roster of things I keep in my head that I know he likes and that I know he'll eat. But I will never say it's vegan, because immediately he's going to dismiss it as something he doesn't like. If I just serve it to him, and ask him, what do you like about it and what don't you like about it, it's a more meaningful conversation. My mom will say, "Oh, let's go to this vegan restaurant." My father will say, "Absolutely not." I'll say, "Alright Dad, don't worry", and I'll bring him there anyway. "This is what we're doing and I'm the one who's driving, so you're my hostage. This is where we're going to eat."

I do compromise. They love The Keg steak house restaurant, and there isn't one near where they live. So we'll go one night to The Keg. But, there is going to be at least one night that we're going to a vegan place. I try to make it a different place every time that they come. My mother doesn't want to leave Toronto until she's had brunch at Fresh, the vegan restaurant. It's one of her favourite things to do in Toronto. It doesn't matter what else she does when she visits, before she leaves, we go for brunch at Fresh.

When you go with your parents to The Keg, how do you manage that?

There's nothing on that menu that we can eat, let's face it, it's a steak house. However, it's amazing what can be done with side dishes. If you look through the salad portion, every salad has meat in it. I will customize. Wow, look, they have a baked potato on this menu item, and they've got steamed green beans on that menu item. I'll ask them to make me a plate of potato and steamed green beans. What are they going to say? No? Of course not, they want repeat business. The reality is that there are more and more vegans these days. Restaurants need to have a game plan for that. It's really my last alternative if there's nothing on a menu. I will customize my meal with side dishes that I've tailored. For example, it's great that the baked potato comes with butter, and sour cream, and cheese, like wow, that sounds delicious. Is there any way I can get it without all that stuff? A lot of places have salsas, and hot sauces or whatever, you can always find something. What restaurant these days, especially in Toronto, does not have hot sauce? I love hot sauce and that would be delicious on that potato.

You mentioned how your co-workers make fun of you for being vegan. How do you handle that?

It's mostly my boss. He will say, "Well, we don't know what we're going to feed Sabina." However, that being said, often the person who comes to pick off my plate at lunch time is my boss. He'll say, "Wow, that's delicious and interesting. How did you make it?" At work, we're all foodies, you know. Wine and food, they just go together.

I'm eating a bigger array of foods than omnivores. They're just eating the same food prepared different ways. There's a whole world of things I had no idea existed. I've learned some really great things. I've learned there's no vegetable that I don't like. Except for maybe okra, but I'll still eat it. We live in the biggest city in Canada and we're so incredibly fortunate to have everything. You name it, you can find it here. If you go to an Asian market, and wonder what the heck that vegetable is, you ask someone and learn something new. You go to farmers' markets, where they love to give you new ideas of what to do with new vegetables.

You said that your doctor was happy with the way you were eating, but since you've undertaken eating *The Starch Solution* way, how is she relating to you now?

We have this running joke over the years that I won't take prescriptions because of my history of being stoned most of my childhood. She was quite happy that I had done enough research and looked at other alternatives. Of course, there's always going to be an issue for most people. Taking medication has its time and place, but I think we're far too reliant on them as a society. If I can avoid it, I do. My doctor doesn't advocate for this way of eating, but she wasn't surprised either with the results. She was nothing but supportive. All of my numbers were exactly where they should be. She made a couple of suggestions. I think I was on the low end for B_{12} and for iron, but still in the normal range. She said eat a few more leafy vegetables and take a higher dose of B_{12}. That was it, because she knows I'm not going to be relying on drugs. She even said that she wished more people would look at their lifestyle and what adjustments they can make rather than just coming here and expecting to be given a medication. The fact that I've taken that extra step and I've looked at it myself instead of having to rely on a doctor, I think she's very supportive of that. I know that a lot of people's doctors are not.

Where is your support coming from? The kind of support that we all need is when you are free to speak your truth.

It's mostly with the group that we've put together, The Toronto Starch Solution Meetup group. I have found more like-minded people. You're not going to change anyone, but you can certainly surround yourself with people who are going to be supportive and lift you up rather than tear you down. That's really become my philosophy. I've been around people who are miserable and destructive. No one really likes to be around that. With the Toronto Starch Solution group, they are people just like me.

With problem-solving, let's say it's a wedding, what would you do?

That's a great question. I try to opt out of those types of events. I mean, most people whose wedding I'd attend already know this about me. If they're at a banquet hall or what not, same thing, they want to accommodate the guests. It's probably not appropriate to bring your own food to something like that, but you can certainly speak with the chef and offer up some recipes or ideas. Give them specific examples, don't just say, "I don't eat meat, and I don't eat dairy or eggs, and I don't eat oil." Say, "These are the things I avoid, but here are the things I do eat, here are some great ideas." Or, you can do what you did at the restaurant. Ask what they're serving. What is everyone else eating? What from those dishes can you take and make your meal vegan? If it's going to be the steak and potatoes, and the green beans, well the potatoes and the green beans are a great start.

If it's a social situation where you're going to someone's home to eat, I usually will offer to bring food. I eat this way and I don't expect anyone else to cook this way, but I would really love the opportunity to bring some things and share with the group. Maybe it's the side dishes that you're going to make. They're going to have what they consider the main event, the carcass on the table, and you can bring everything else that they would call side dishes. First, you're going to eat really, really well. Second, so are the other people at the event. Third, wow, this is vegan?! It's a really great conversation starter. Often, I'm asked how I made the dish I've brought, and it's great to share something positive with other people.

Do you have any advice for beginners?

Keep it simple, as simple as possible. Don't worry about these odd ingredients. If you don't know what nutritional yeast is, don't worry about it. Stick to things that you're already eating, that are familiar to you. Everybody knows how to cook a potato. Great! But why not look at your roster. People tend to rotate through the same meals, week after week. Look at some of your favorites and how you can veganize them. Chili is a great one. It's easy to just keep meat out of it, and maybe add another type of bean or lentils or something to fill it out. Those are easy switches to make.

Speaking of chili, please share your story about the wedding reception and the food you brought.

Oh, yes, that's a great story. A friend of mine was married in New Zealand, and they decided to have a party in Canada. What they did, rather than a traditional reception, is they did it as a potluck. They know that I'm vegan. I should mention that the groom is a chef. I showed up with my big Instant Pot of vegan chili and a cornbread that I had made. I didn't say anything. I just plugged in my Instant Pot to keep it warm. Well, there was not a morsel left behind, I mean the whole thing was gone. The bride asked "Did everyone enjoy the chili? By the way, it was vegan." The people were beside themselves. There's no way that was vegan, it was delicious. How on earth…? There was meat in there! No, there wasn't. And guess what, I didn't put any fake meat in either. I added some red lentils to really fill it out and make it heavy, as though there was meat in it. People think they can't get full on vegan food. People were coming and asking, "Oh but the cornbread wasn't vegan, was it?" It absolutely was vegan. They said, "How on earth?" And by the way, there was no oil. "That's impossible! What did you use instead of oil?" I used applesauce. "You can do that?" Absolutely, who says you can't? The comments included the chef husband who said, "Oh wow, that was great." It was that leading by example thing.

What can you do now, that you couldn't do before you started *The Starch Solution*?

I think I'm more self-assertive, I have more confidence. I'm not so concerned anymore about what others think of me being vegan. Since meeting the group, I'm not hiding the fact that I'm vegan anymore. I'm a lot more confident about saying, "Yes, this is what I eat and this is what I don't eat." I've been positively surprised that more and more people are positive about it, or inquisitive, rather than immediately negative.

How has this way of eating impacted your mood?

My mood is so much better and lighter. I think in general, eating this way, it doesn't bring you down. I remember back when I would have a Thanksgiving meal with turkey and all of that, and lots of dairy, you would feel heavy. You would have to shut down and go sleep or something. Now, rather than just being lethargic, food is doing what it was intended to do. It's giving me energy. I'm much clearer headed and enthusiastic. It's like you have this surplus of energy you need to burn off rather than just going home, plopping yourself on the sofa, and watching TV as you fall asleep because you can't do anything else.

I mean, look at animals in the wild that do eat meat as part of their diet. Lions, what do they do after eating, they sleep for two days! It's because their bodies are working so hard to digest, even though lions are meant to eat that. For us humans, even though we can get away with eating meat, it doesn't mean that we should. Our bodies must work overtime in trying to neutralize that sort of stuff. When you stop eating it, you realize, wow, I feel really great.

How has it affected you spiritually?

I'm not religious but I think I'm spiritual. This has put to the forefront that everything is connected. Everyone is connected, not just people but the planet, animals, everything is connected and we all rely on each other. I think it's to do with the pagan religions and Wicca. There's a great expression they have, "Harm none." I think it's a wonderful way to think about it. Their philosophy is that if you inflict harm, it's going to come back to you threefold. I think that is what we're experiencing now. If you look at the planet, the ecology, the environment, and our health, it's affecting us in a negative way. I think that just comes back to having a full understanding of spirituality, that we're all connected. It's in our best interest to preserve everything we can. Don't be cruel to people. We don't need religion to tell us to be decent human beings. As we know, people will use religion to further their own causes, be it positive or not. I think spirituality is a step further.

Do you notice a shift in how your mind works, as in clarity of thought, and the ability to grasp complex issues?

Yes, it has increased exponentially. I'm a lot clearer in my thoughts. It gives me the ability to put more energy to working out complex ideas in my head. Be it for my job or personally. I don't get so exhausted and decide not to resolve something. Oh, I'll deal with it later. It gives me the ability to look at things that are more complex and make them more straightforward so that I understand them. I'm an information junkie. I love, love, love to learn about things. There are a lot of complicated things in this world, and I feel I'm better equipped to wrap my head around foreign concepts and complex things than I could before.

There's been a lot said about the impact of a whole food plant-based diet, or vegan lifestyle, on the environment and animal rights. What are your thoughts?

Similar to my answer about spirituality, it's all connected. Treat others the way you would like to be treated. I'm pretty darn sure we wouldn't want to be barred away, force fed things, and ultimately slaughtered. I mean, it's ingrained. Every human, every animal, wants to preserve their life. No one wants to have their life ended and that includes other beings on this planet. I don't care if you're a pig, a shark, or a human. We all are programmed to survive. Just because we are able to enforce our will onto others doesn't make it right.

As a result, we're killing the planet as well. The United Nations have a stat that 51 percent of all greenhouse gases come from animal agriculture. That's more than half! I don't care if you drive a hybrid, you're still partaking in all of these other things. You're really contributing to the problem, in fact, you're a big part of the problem.

There's this great documentary, *Cowspiracy*, where the person doing the documentary wanted to interview some environmental organizations. The top of his list was Greenpeace, who refused to talk to him because he wanted to talk about animal agriculture. Yet, you talk about Greenpeace being this amazing environmental organization, and what do they talk about when you go to their website. Well, it's the car that you drive, and so on. It's great that people are making those changes, but it's not enough.

We have completely ravaged the oceans to where it may not come back at this point. We've knocked out entire species because that's what I feel like eating tonight. It's so ridiculously selfish. Ecology-wise, and for the ethics of how we use animals, we shouldn't be using animals at all. We have no business in doing that.

Do you have any further goals related to diet and exercise?

I want to do things that are fun. I'm spending more time outside, going out for walks, and having little adventures in my neighborhood. I know my neighborhood like the back of my hand driving, but how often do I just go out and find these little side streets that wouldn't take me anywhere. There might be a dead end, you know. It's more about going out and enjoying what we have around us. I mean, how unnatural is it to go somewhere and get on a machine to get your exercise. Why not go out and walk? Or swim, I love to swim. Do what feels good. For me, I spent so much time in hibernation. I grew up in Northern Ontario where it feels like perpetual winter sometimes. The last thing you ever want to do is go outside. I live in Toronto now, and yes, we've had some hard winters but not like where I grew up. There's no reason for me to not be spending more time outside. I'm doing things that are just fun.

Next summer I've signed up to do slow-pitch baseball. It's once or twice a week, with a team. I've never done that sort of thing before. I'm not athletic or into organized sports. But guess what, neither are any of these people. It's just about getting together and doing something that's good for your health and having fun at the same time. Maybe meet some new people. I'm trying to focus more on doing things like that rather than spending a good amount of money on something that kind of makes me miserable.

Tell me about your career goals since becoming vegan.

I've been fantasizing about putting together a talk and educating people to understand if the wine they're looking at is safe for vegans. A lot of people don't know that three very popular ingredients that are added to wines are fish bladders, egg whites, and casein, which is the protein from cow's milk. These are things plant-based people are trying to avoid, but if you like to drink wine, how do you know whether these things were used in the making of the wine you've just purchased? How do you tell the difference? I would talk about labelling, say in Canada, which has been progressive in this area, versus the United States. If you're interested in a wine, you'll want to know what questions to be asking. What are the alternatives? Even talking to people about what does it mean to be sustainable versus a natural wine, versus organic, or biodynamic. It really goes back to this whole idea that everything is connected. Wine is an agricultural product. A lot of people, wine consumers, they forget that. Even spirit producers do. Vodkas, whiskeys, and rum, we're talking about things coming from plants. Vodka can be made from almost anything, potatoes, grains, and whatever else, rum from sugar cane and whiskey from grains.

What are your overall life goals? Are they different from what they were before you became vegan?

I would say that before I became vegan, I didn't have a goal. I was in a fog that only people who have become vegan understand. When you get clarity of mind, suddenly, it gives you the opportunity to look at your life. You've changed this thing in your life. It gives you the chance to say, wait a minute, there is something else out there. It gave me an opportunity to consider what I thought was important. How am I going to live a meaningful life that's going to be meaningful for me, not for anyone else. Having that clarity, it brought me to this position of what I want to do with my career and in educating people. If I had the ideal lifestyle, I would love to just be able to travel the world and talk to people about this sort of thing. I'd extend it into food because I always tell people that wine is just liquid food. It kind of goes together. It's important to know where these things come from and how they're produced. When things are not in line with those values, not to give them the financial backing to continue what they're doing.

I've been fortunate to work with several artisanal producers who are making phenomenal products, just working the land, and working with Mother Nature rather than trying to work against her. They understand that everything is connected. It all comes back to that. What you do to the land is going to end up in the water, and ultimately will end up in your glass. You really need to be careful of what you're doing. Sadly, it's mainly smaller producers that are doing this, but because of this whole revolution we're having in the world of ecology, and things that are more front of mind, people are asking the questions. Some of the big guys are starting to respond, making sure they're going to start producing better products. Of course, there will be people who will argue against me, but overall, the more attention and the better fruit you produce, the better your product. It all comes from the land. Any farmer is going to tell you, it comes from the soil.

Do you have the desire to be more involved with environmental and/or animal activism?

Yes, I do. In the past year, I visited a farm sanctuary for the first time, which was a wonderful experience. It really was. I'd like to do more of that. I visited one near my parents' home and brought my mom and dad with me. They had a great day. It was a fundraiser they were having. We went out and saw some animals, and had one goat that was very excited to meet us and wanted to be petted.

In terms of activism, I'm very supportive and grateful for anyone who does any type of animal activism. One of my favorites on the planet is the Sea Shepherd Conservation Society. I think Captain Paul Watson is doing some amazing stuff. He's inspiring. Am I going to throw myself in the front lines? I'd like to think I'm that kind of person, and I do know people like that and I admire these people so much. I think we need these people. People say, "Oh, what about these things PETA does, it's not so great." I say, "You know, nobody was even touching this subject until PETA came on the scene. They've really pushed that conversation forward and I'm so incredibly grateful." I was introduced to veganism by PETA. I support these organizations and I fantasize sometimes, "Oh, maybe I'll volunteer on one of these Sea Shepherd campaigns." I don't know if I have that in me, but I'd love to think that I do. I try to support them anytime I see them anywhere. I drop by their booths, I do what I can. Yeah, maybe one day I'll be one of those people, hanging off a billboard and getting arrested for causing a nuisance. We'll see.

I'm a communicator. I'm a marketer. I'm happy to help promote and push forward that message. Maybe one day, I will be that crazy person, but that hasn't happened yet. I'm not quite comfortable with hanging out naked on the sidewalk, just with body paint, as some of the PETA people do. It's phenomenal. I must say, I always kind of rolled my eyes when I saw that online. Then, they did it in Toronto where I almost tripped over these two women outside the Eaton's Centre in downtown Toronto. They were covered with pieces of produce and then I saw they were with PETA. I thought, "This is phenomenal." It was one of the best things I've ever seen in my life. I would never have the courage to do that. By the way, aren't these attractive ladies? They're vegan!

You talk to most meat-loving men, and when it comes to sexual relations, they're very happy to be with a vegan woman. Because, we vegans, we don't smell.

That's right! People think I'm crazy when I say that, but it's true. Plus, everything is running optimally. Therefore, the scents are not the same. There's this expression that comes from the Asian culture, it's an expression that's starting to fall by the way side. Asians used to say that Westerners had a stink to them because they were dairy eaters. For a long time in the Asian cultures, there was no dairy consumption at all. They could smell the Westerners a mile away.

You know, people have often said, "You're all for the animals, what about humans?" You know what, ultimately, we vegans are also trying to help the human race by promoting the messages that we are. There's this documentary called *Unsupersize* Me. This woman, dealing with obesity and other health problems, was put on a plant-based diet. One of the first realizations she made was the need for meat to be in separate bags, since meat would contaminate other foods if it were to be in contact with them. Oh, my God, meat is contaminating! She literally made that shift on camera. If this is contaminating everything else then maybe I shouldn't be eating meat.

Dr. Michael Greger has a video on his nutritionfacts.org website, where he talks about people who clean chicken in their kitchen sinks or on their counters, and will have bacteria from the chicken that takes five days to clear up. These bacteria are resistant to cleaning. That means most kitchens have bacteria lurking on the counter and in the sink, and no amount of anti-bacterial cleaners and scrubbing will get rid of them.

What about the Paleo diet advocates?

It's just Atkins re-packaged, as far as I'm concerned. I'm sure there's a lot of agro-business behind the Paleo craze because now it's Paleo everything. I think it's awful, but there is one positive. At least, they're promoting whole foods; they just haven't gone far enough. I still think it's dangerous. The Paleo diet has never reversed heart disease, for example.

When you went vegan, did you find that for the first couple of weeks, your BMs were horrible, really smelly?

Yes, that's right, I remember that. That was years of impacted meats that had been stuck in my intestines and were finally able to clear out. That is the most common thing I hear from people who have gone plant-based. Plus, there's little to no smell now. Chef AJ said that your body becomes this amazing digestion machine. Things just run smoothly, the way they're supposed to. I had digestive issues from adolescence. Now, I have zero problems.

Anything else you feel is important to share?

I think we're not all in that same mindset. No matter what, be compassionate with people and hopefully that will be reciprocal. Be understanding, kill 'em with kindness. Be willing to laugh and to smile and to be really kind to people. People who can be cruel and close minded may realize "I'm being a jerk right now", this person's just being kind and nice.

Be as nice as you possibly can, but don't let people walk all over you, of course. We don't know other people's stories, they don't know our stories. Maybe it's stemming from something, and it's got nothing to do with us, so just try to be understanding and compassionate. Lead by example. Don't be afraid to speak your own truth, and I have to believe that is going to make all the difference in the world.

Chapter Fourteen
Judith

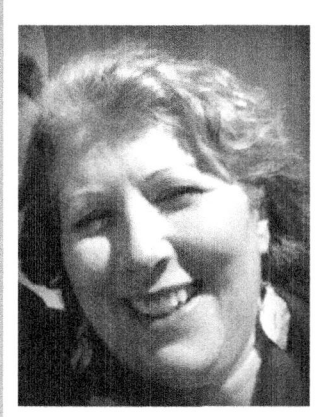

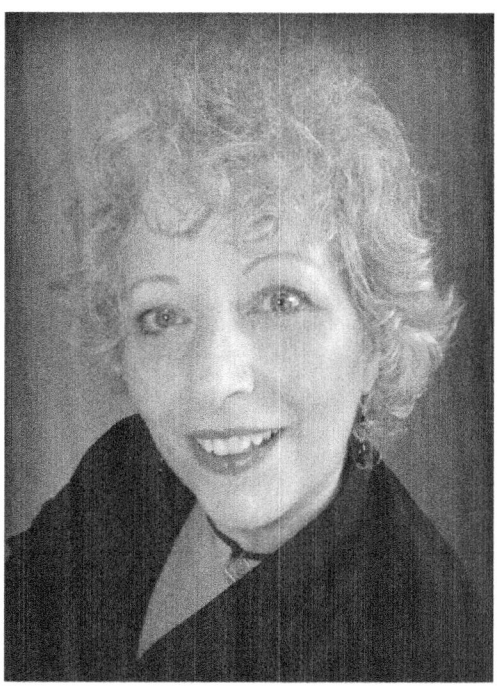

Judith's cholesterol and blood pressure were climbing, and her obesity was out of control. Out of the blue, she was struck with pericarditis that compromised her heart function and landed her in the hospital. Here is Judith's inspiring story of recovering her optimal health, which so far includes a weight loss of 65 pounds.

Chapter Fourteen - Judith's Interview

Tell us a bit about yourself.

I'm a naturopathic doctor, in practice now for over 17 years. My focus is primarily fertility, and I mainly offer nutritional support and acupuncture treatment. I've been married for 29 years, and my husband Dom and I have two grown children, a son and a daughter. We also have a Jack Russell Terrier named Lulu. I think it's important to mention her because she's my personal trainer; she gets me out for daily walks.

Please tell us your personal story relative to Dr. McDougall's program *The Starch Solution.*

I didn't start following Dr. McDougall's *Starch Solution* program until June of 2015. Before that, back in December of 2011, I had gone to see my doctor. I had gained more weight and he said, "You know you're pushing 300 pounds here". I think I was 298 pounds at the time. I said, "I'll work on a diet." However, this is December. It's Christmas time. Not a great time to think about dieting. My doctor said, "You're pre-diabetic, and your cholesterol levels are high." He also said, "Given your weight, it's understandable. I'm going to have to start you on medication." For me, that set off alarm bells and I asked him for time to change things, to lose some weight, and lower my cholesterol that way. He agreed to give me six months. If I were to lose weight and lower my cholesterol and blood sugars on my own, then he wouldn't be prescribing me any drugs.

So of course, Christmas came and I went to town with the food. I ate everything in sight. I knew I would start the diet in January and I decided I would have one last "hurrah" of all the treats I loved to eat. Finally, Christmas was done. I remember it was January 2nd, and I got on the scale and it said 308 pounds. While I wasn't surprised, with the way I had been eating for the last couple of weeks, it was still a devastating moment for me. Never in my life did I think I would go over 300 pounds.

I had been doing research and I decided to give up dairy. I was looking at all the fat in dairy and all the calories, and I knew I was a cheese addict. Cheese was always my "go to" snack, and it was the best thing I did, to eliminate dairy from my life. My research also brought me to this lecture by Gary Yourofsky. In the lecture, he was talking about being 100 percent vegan for the animals. He showed a video of this guy on a dairy farm and he was horribly abusing the cows and the baby calves. I was crying when I was watching this. That really helped me to go completely dairy-free and it also made my resolve very strong to start into plant-based eating.

I had toyed with being vegan several years before and I remember I felt sort of okay, but I wasn't doing it right. I wasn't concerned about proper nutrients. I didn't eat meat, fish, dairy, and eggs, but I was still eating tons of sugar. I was still eating cookies, granola bars, and rice milk ice cream. I was still eating a lot of junk. Basically, I was a junk food vegan, so it's no wonder why I didn't feel that great. This time, I decided to focus on nutrition and eat healthier foods. I realized that for me, it would be best to ease my way into more plant-based eating. I started off with eating 100 percent plant-based Monday to Friday, and on weekends I allowed myself to have small portions of beef, chicken, and fish. By the end of March, I got on the scale and I was 286 pounds. Just by dropping dairy and eating plant-based five days out of seven, I had lost 22 pounds. I thought that was really good.

On Sunday April 29th, 2012, my daughter and I went out for brunch. I ate two poached eggs with toast, and I had one piece of bacon from my daughter's plate. I came out of that restaurant and I could barely walk to my car. It was like I'd just been run over by a Mack truck. The air was molasses and I couldn't move very well. My daughter asked what was wrong, and I said "Sweetie, I cannot do this anymore."

The minute we got home, I went back to watching the lecture with Gary Yourofsky. My daughter asked to watch it with me. I warned her about the animal abuse, but at 17 years old, she felt she could handle it. My daughter became vegan right at that moment when she watched that video. Up until then, she had observed me eating more plant-based and she thought that was great. When she watched that video she said, "Mom, I am doing this too" and she has - she amazes me. She hasn't looked back since then.

Along with my daughter, I became strictly plant-based on Sunday, April 29th, 2012. I wasn't following Dr. McDougall's plan yet, I was still eating oil. My weight had settled into a range of 270 to 280 pounds. Not great, but at least not 308 pounds.

My next visit to my doctor went really well. My cholesterol had dropped and I was no longer pre-diabetic. The doctor was pleased with my weight loss, but he still thought I would need to have bariatric surgery. That was it, I just never made another appointment to see this doctor. I knew my health wasn't exactly stellar, even with eating plant-based. Even though I was having lots of greens and fruits, all healthy foods like that, the oil, salt, and sugar still figured prominently. I think I'm addicted to those foods, to be honest.

Then, in the summer of 2014, I started having chest pain. I went to the ER, and was diagnosed with viral pericarditis. For 98 percent of people with that diagnosis, a two-week round of high-dose ibuprofen will take care of it. However, I was in the two percent who go on to have the pericardium (it's the sac or lining that the heart sits in) fill with fluid, to the point where my heart couldn't function very well. Basically, it's like heart failure, and that is not a great thing at all. If I tried to lie down I couldn't breathe, and my blood pressure would crash and I'd nearly pass out.

I went to the hospital via ambulance. My blood pressure was going up and down, and I was having episodes of gasping for breath. In the ER, I heard the doctor say to the nurse on the other side of the curtain, "She doesn't look very good." That's not a comforting thing to hear from an ER doc, and I wondered if I was dying. (I found out later that there are deaths due to severe pericarditis. Eventually, the heart stops.) Fortunately, once my blood pressure was stabilized with IV fluids, I was able to have the surgery to drain the fluid out from around my heart.

It took me nearly 18 months to fully recover. I had to return to the hospital two more times. The lining of my left lung was filling with fluid and I needed a lung tap to drain it. Then, another time my chest pain was returning and the echo (ultrasound) on my heart showed there was a bit of fluid. There was also some fluid forming in the lining of my right lung. The ibuprofen had never worked for me, so I was prescribed Indomethacin, and for me it was a miracle drug because it cleared up all of the fluids. My cardiologist didn't want me to stay on it for more than a few weeks, however, and I knew I had to find a way to keep the inflammation at bay.

It was inflammation that was causing all of my problems, and I had to figure out what to do about it. One thing I noticed was that if I ate oils and fats like vegan margarine, I could feel a kind of electric heat in the right side of my chest. I realized that was the beginning sign of inflammation. That electric heat feeling was my warning. I have to say, I'm very grateful I had that sensation. It started to teach me that I felt best with plain vegetables and whole foods.

I went online in March of 2015 and I saw a lot of success stories on Dr. McDougall's site. I bought his book, *The Starch Solution*. I was beside myself with joy because I didn't want to give up potatoes and rice. All the other diets are saying, "Oh no-no-no, limit your carbs. Don't have them. It's so fattening." But nobody was saying stop the oil. "Oh no-no-no, you need fats, they are healthy for us." Get the oils, get the nuts, the seeds, and so on and so forth. By the time I came to doing Dr. McDougall's plan, my weight had climbed up again. I was about 285 pounds. Like Dr. McDougall says, "The fat you eat is the fat you wear."

I was on the McDougall forum, searching for other people in Toronto that I could meet with face-to-face. I ended up connecting with Judy and Kathy, who have both had remarkable changes in their health and well-being. We went out for tea, and we decided to start a Meetup group. We decided to call it the Toronto Starch Solution Meetup Group. We wanted to be very specific about what kind of plant-based eating we were doing. A lot of people don't want to say starch, or don't believe that eating starch will help them to lose weight and get healthy. But we wanted it clearly spelled out what kind of group we are, and that this is how we are eating. There are a lot of vegan meetup groups but they still include a lot of fat and sugar in their diet. I don't think it's healthy. After all, I was eating that way and my weight was increasing.

I still struggle. I think oil is a gateway food that leads me to my addiction to sugar and flour. As long as I avoid oil, I don't get the cravings for pasta and pancakes. Seriously, I could eat pasta and pancakes all day. I can stay away from oil at least 80 percent of the time. The issue is I live in a household where potato chips and olive oil are front and center. It's a part of my environment.

My most difficult time of the year is from October to Christmas. Things can get out of control because between mid-October to December I have the following events: Thanksgiving, my daughter's birthday, my wedding anniversary, my husband's birthday, my birthday and Christmas. There's a lot of celebrating going on, with a lot of high fat vegan foods. In spite of those birthdays and holidays, I am learning how to get right back on plan. One of the best things I've found is to follow Chef AJ's advice and eat a huge salad for breakfast the very next day after a celebration. The only dressing I use is a bit of balsamic vinegar. It's really delicious and I feel really great. The cravings go away when I eat that salad for breakfast. When I'm focused on weight loss, the breakfast salad helps me stay on track quite well.

I've got John McDougall's other book, *The McDougall Program for Maximum Weight Loss*, so I know what I have to do. There is no kidding around. I know it's no nuts, no refined carbohydrates like flour, no oils, no margarine or vegan butter, no avocados, no tofu, no seeds, no extraneous fats of any kind. I follow the MWL (Maximum Weight Loss) plan at least 80 to 90 percent now, and it works for me. I am continuing to lose weight and feel better.

Who else has inspired you along the way besides Dr. McDougall?

Pretty well all of them. Dr. Caldwell Esselstyn, Jeff Novick, and Chef AJ come to mind. Since the Remedy seminar in Toronto, Brenda Davis has become a real inspiration. I was very impressed with her. Then, of course, Dr. Neal Barnard is a big favorite. I also admire Dr. T. Colin Campbell a great deal. It was his book *The China Study* that first opened up my eyes to the health benefits of plant-based eating. Cancer, stroke and Alzheimer's are the ones that are very prevalent in my family history. Hopefully I can put off Alzheimer's, maybe never get it, and never have to deal with stroke and cancer. I want to get old and wear out and drift off. I would like to live to be at least 90. My grandmother lived to be 98, but she suffered with Alzheimer's for years. I remember the last years of her life. She was tied into a chair because otherwise, she would fall out. She was in diapers, of course. She couldn't really speak. She'd watch the TV and kind of smile at it, but if you fed her candy then she really loved you. She'd smile and laugh. She couldn't recognize anybody anymore. My poor grandmother, she didn't know anybody at the end.

How has this diet changed your life?

It has given me hope. It's allowing me to think that I have a future, even at my age of 58. I am not done yet. I also hope that I can finally get to a normal body weight like I was in my 20s before I had kids. You know, my weight when I was in my 20s ranged from 125 to 130 pounds. I don't expect to be that small again (although it would be amazing if I could), but if I could get down to somewhere around 140 to 150 pounds, that would be a good weight for me. That would be exciting. It's happening. This program is the means.

This meetup has brought a whole new set of friends in my life. As you get older, you need to make new friends. Old friends seem to drift off and you get compartmentalized. With older people in their 60s to 80s who are in failing health, it's really hard for them to connect with new people. Their spouses have passed on or they're divorced and they get isolated and lonely. Even if your kids are really close to you, they still have their own lives to get on with. I think this is a big reason why I have my dog Lulu. If I didn't have Lulu, I'd be so lonely. Nothing against my husband, but he has his friends that he hangs out with down at the coffee bar or the market, or buddies through acting. In my profession as a naturopathic doctor, it's a one-person business and I am on my own. It gets lonely.

What have been your main obstacles?

The main one is the belief that I would never have a shot at getting to a normal size again. In the past, when I'd eat a little bit of something I knew I shouldn't be eating, I'd think, "Oh God I'm cheating." My mind would go to that dark place, thinking I can never get slim and that I will always be fat. Now, with the way I am eating I'm not craving all those crappy foods. Now, I can walk past a bakery and I look at the stuff in the window and it's almost like looking at plastic figurines. It looks very pretty but I am not interested in eating it. When I look at a plate of brownies now, I get grossed out. I am really grossed out at the amount of sugar and fat that is in those things. It just disgusts me. This is a good place to be.

What kind of issues have come up with your family and friends?

With friends, I am sure I have lost one friendship over me eating plant-based. I am sure she got fed up from hearing how eating meat and dairy is a problem. I tried to get together with her, sent emails and she never replied. I haven't heard from her since and that feels quite sad. I realize I was going on a lot about eating plant-based and how great the health benefits were, and I guess she didn't want to hear it. I was a new convert and I thought because we were friends, I could be up front with her and share my excitement. I have to remind myself that nobody likes a zealot. I've learned to tone things down a lot since then and haven't had any problems with other friends.

With my family, I've made it clear that our kitchen is vegan. I'm fortunate that my daughter is vegan and that my husband is 100 percent on board with only making plant-based meals at home. He enjoys the food. He loves vegetables, thank God! However, he's Italian and olive oil is like air to him. Lately, it's been a lot better. When he cooks, he no longer puts oil in the food. He's water frying or roasting things in the oven on a pan lined with parchment paper. That is a big change and I'm grateful that he's doing that.

What has helped is that he's also given up dairy and his reflux is gone. He was having difficulty sleeping with the reflux and now, it's no longer a problem. My son who is away at university isn't plant-based. He knows that when he comes home for a visit, it's all vegan all the time. If he wants some meat, I tell him he's got the barbecue out in the backyard and he's welcome to cook up a bit of meat if that's what he wants.

What is exciting though, is that in his apartment, he cooks almost 100 percent plant-based for himself. When he's out with friends, he'll eat chicken or burgers, but in his apartment he's making chickpea stew with lots of vegetables, or meatless chili with brown rice. He's studying to be a registered nurse, and I think his exposure to healthcare is helping him be more aware of how best to nourish himself.

Also, he just watched the film *What the Health* on Netflix with a friend, and the two of them have gone vegan for 30 days. He doubts he'll stick with it after the end of the month, but he thinks he'll eat more plant-based because of it. He does say he's hungry all the time, and I tell him to eat lots of potatoes!

What about your doctor? Is he on board with these changes and how has he been relating to you about the food?

There are two doctors to talk about. There is my new GP. I've been with him for about a year. Since my last visit, he's been pushing me to have bariatric surgery and I really don't want to do that. There are studies showing problems with nutrient uptake and so on. He believes that taking some extra vitamins is a lot better than having to deal with heart disease, cancer, and diabetes. I get that, he's recommending what he thinks is best for me, his patient. I like him though, mainly because he does support a vegan diet. He's a young doctor and he's cool with what the research says. I will be seeing him again in about six months, and my plan is to walk in there at least 40 pounds lighter. Hopefully the bariatric surgery idea will no longer be mentioned!

The other doctor is my cardiologist. I love my cardiologist. He is just a sweet, nice guy. He listens and he is good with negotiating with me. He knows I won't do it unless the research clearly shows benefits. He tried to get me to take a beta blocker when I was already on a blood pressure pill. I said, "Nope, nope, won't do that. I know what road I'm going down. Next thing I'll be on is diuretics. No, no, no, no, no, I'm not going there." He worked with me when I changed my diet and it was great to go off the blood pressure medication. He was happy with my changes. He is open to this way of eating. I think he's impressed that my blood pressure has normalized without medication, just an oil-free, starch-based way of eating.

In fact, it is common knowledge in the field of cardiac care that eating a low-fat plant-based diet will have dramatic effects. They all know it but they won't tell their patients because they believe that patients won't change their diets. Why? Because doctors don't have the time to go through nutrition, and more importantly, most medical doctors have very little knowledge of nutrition. Plus, people are emotionally attached to their food. Einstein was quoted as saying that it's easier for a man to change his religion than to change his diet. I think that's why doctors don't mention trying diet. I just wish doctors were more informed and could at least give their patients the information. It could save a lot of lives.

Where is your support coming from now?

Primarily, from our Toronto Starch Solution Meetup group. I think it's important to connect with other people doing the same kind of eating plan as you. It's vital to surround yourself with like-minded people who really get you and can be there to catch you if you are struggling. The YouTube videos of all the different talks given by the plant-based docs are helpful. I especially love the success stories on Dr. McDougall's website. They're so inspiring and there are so many of them. It's awesome.

How do you manage your food when you're out at social events like weddings, parties, and barbecues?

I bring my own food to parties, barbecues, and other social events. I haven't had to deal with a wedding yet but I am fine with bringing my own food. Seriously, I don't care anymore. My life and my health are too important to me. I'm honest with people. I say, "I'm whole food plant-based with no oil." They say, "Oh, I can't begin to figure out how to feed you." I say, "Not to worry, I'll feed myself and I'll bring enough for everybody to sample." If I happen to get resistance (which is rare), then I will add that I'm on doctor's orders and that's why I have to bring my own food. (The doctor I'm referring to is Dr. McDougall, of course!)

The thing is, for any social event, you do what you have to do. If you're on vacation or eating out in restaurants all the time, you do what you have to do. If you are in a new place, call around to vegan and vegetarian restaurants. Some will probably know what you mean when you say "I'm a McDougaller. I can't have oil, doctor's orders. What can you do for me?" Another idea is to travel around with your Instant Pot like Chef AJ does. She has a whole YouTube video on how she travels. It's amazing.

Do you have any advice for beginners?

It is going to take some time. Ask yourself, are you an all or nothing type of person? Can you jump in 100 percent no problem? Or are you someone that has to ease your way into it? If you have to ease your way in, then you can start out like I did. For example, just quit dairy. That is a big source of addiction for most people and if you can start with no dairy, it's going to make a huge difference in your health and how you feel. Then you can go plant-based at least four days out of seven. I went five days out of seven, doing plant-based Monday to Friday. Eventually, you'll probably find that the days you're eating animal foods are not so great. You'll probably feel bloated or tired. That's when you can do plant-based 100 percent. However, if you're someone who is possibly one meal away from a major heart attack or stroke, then I'd urge you to jump in 100 percent right from the get go. It's your choice, but this is life or death now. Just do it. If you want to keep it simple, go and buy a big sack of potatoes, several cans of beans and bags of frozen vegetables and lots of limes and lemons and that is all you eat for the whole week. Just do it!

I'd also say beware of copping out, of thinking that this is just too hard. If your health is going down the tubes, then you've got to do something about it. You've got to change your diet. The doctors aren't going to do that for you, only you can do it. When I hear someone who keeps complaining about their health, but who refuses to change their lifestyle, after awhile, I stop listening to them. It's like someone who won't put a lock on their front door, but they're complaining about the intruders who come in to rob them and beat them up. Helloooooo, put a lock on the door! Same thing with lifestyle, stop complaining about your health and do something. Eat a no-oil, starch-based diet. It works. It's that lock on your front door that's keeping disease and pain out. Isn't that what you want, to be healthy, to not be in pain?

What can you do now that you couldn't do before?

A little over two years ago, I could barely walk a block without feeling awful. I couldn't walk upstairs in my house without getting winded. Now, I can walk up and down my stairs without a thought. I can also walk for an hour at a good pace and still feel great. I had no energy for exercise before. Especially, in the last couple of months of committing to primarily no-oil eating, my energy has been going up. Every day I am feeling better.

How has this way of eating impacted your mood?

Before, I'd get into some bad moods from time to time. I would feel very blue. I'd feel hopeless, helpless, that sort of thing. I'd just have thoughts of, "Why bother? I'm never going to get healthy again. I'm just going to continue to decline." I was really down about it all. Now, with the physical changes, my mood is phenomenal. I have hope. I look forward to the future. I am making plans. I had stopped making plans when I was sick. Now, I'm making plans and I've never been happier.

What kind of plans?

I'm making plans that are about this book we are writing, of course. I'm also planning to write another book, based on the success I'm having with my fertility patients. I'm calling it *Plant Powered Procreation*. I'm looking forward to helping as many people as possible, to help them discover how much better they can be.

How about energy level?

I feel fabulous. I can move my body! I have to share with you a passage from *The Starch Solution*, when Dr. McDougall talks about how your friends are going to be pretty jealous of how much better you're feeling and looking. How they won't be able to keep up with you on a walk, that sort of thing. That's what is happening for me. My energy is fabulous. I am getting better and better every day.

Have you noticed a difference in your attitude?

I am a lot calmer. I am a lot easier going. I am much less likely to get in a tizzy about things. I'll still have a little thing here and there that sort of ruffles my feathers. But overall, I am a lot more open and forgiving, calm and spiritual. I don't know how else to describe it. It just feels so good.

Have you noticed a shift in how your mind has been working?

Yes, I do. I am finding now that I can read some very technical and complicated information and easily grasp it. A lot of what I read is scientific studies, because as a naturopath I often have to do some research before making recommendations for my patients. I am finding I'm able to go through a study and very quickly be able to pick up what it's all about, whereas before I'd have to kind of slog through it.

There has been a lot said about the impact of a whole food plant-based diet or vegan lifestyle on the environment and animal rights. What are your thoughts?

I can't even begin to comprehend the horror of what animals are going through every time they're pushed onto the slaughterhouse floor and there's blood and death and murder all around them. People are eating their meat, ingesting the terror of their final moments. In a spiritual sense, it is no wonder people are more focused on hatred and putting up walls. How can you invite love and compassion into your heart when you've just eaten the meat from a cow that died a violent death?

The other thing is the environment. If we want half a chance of our human race being able to survive beyond the next fifty years then we have to change. We have to stop eating animals, or at least eat a lot fewer animals. All the billions of animals that we have bred into existence for food that we don't need are contributing to 51 percent of the greenhouse gases and are fueling climate change - just stop eating animals, or at least limit your meat consumption to a maximum of three meals per week. If everybody did that, the impact would be huge for the environment and human health.

I think, with all the evidence we have from the scientific studies done, we can no longer say meat is good for us. The science doesn't support that. The science is clearly showing that we have done this to ourselves. If we want our children and grandchildren to have a shot at being able to survive beyond the next fifty years, then it's time to stop eating animal foods. If we keep going the way we are, then by 2050, it's being predicted there will be no more drinking water left. There will be no fish in the oceans either because the oceans will have become extremely acidic.

The idea that clearing out more and more acreage in the rainforest is okay because, after all, we're planting a few more trees over here, makes no sense to me. That's like have your stomach slashed open, your guts are spilling out, and you're reaching for those finger-sized bandages. It's just not going to work.

I would like to see an end to factory farming. There are a number of viral illnesses that develop in those places, such as avian flu and swine flu, because the animals are in really horrible conditions and their immune systems shut down. It's a field day for these viruses, and we're going to see more of them infecting people. It's a terrible situation for both people and animals. Instead, I would love to see the factory farms turned into huge greenhouse gardens. All the people that have been employed in that industry could now make a living growing beautiful vegetables like corn, beans, potatoes, tomatoes, carrots, lettuces, and everything you can think of. They could plant fruit trees and grow more fruit. I'd rather have more fruit than more viruses.

You know what they did in Denmark? They put it together a long time ago that dairy and meat causes heart disease and illness. They subsidized their farmers to stop raising beef and to grow blueberries.

I'd rather eat blueberries than beef, that's for sure! The problem is that even though people know that eating meat and dairy is the cause of heart disease, they are still going to eat those foods because they say, "Oh well, until I actually get sick I'm not going to worry about it. Besides, meat tastes really good, so why should I stop eating it." People are naturally inclined to be hedonistic and want to have it all and fit as much pleasure as they can while minimizing their pain. Unfortunately, for our environment and our health, that just isn't going to cut it.

Many people choose to ignore the plight of the animals because they don't want to give up the pleasure they derive from eating steak. They keep themselves in the dark. They turn away from the sight of an animal in distress because human beings don't have that inclination towards blood lust. You don't see people driving down the highway and shouting, "Look! Road kill! Let's stop and have a bite!" No, we don't do that. We are disgusted by it because we do not have blood lust. Look at our teeth. Look at our hands. Our teeth and our hands are perfect for plucking fruit from the trees and biting into apples. We are not meant to rip open the hide of a gentle sweet cow or goat and dig in and eat their guts and everything because that is what a true carnivore does.

That is the thing, we humans are so selfish and we often think just about this moment, and the short-term future. We've got to realize that it is not just us. It is our children and our grandchildren. It is our legacy that is totally threatened by us continuing to eat this way and have this kind of lifestyle.

Our carbon footprint is reduced by 70 percent if we go vegan - that is huge! If we did that, we could slow things down, maybe to the point where the human species could live one hundred years beyond that. I think that eventually we are going to go extinct. We are headed on that path, but if we could just give ourselves some more time, who knows, maybe we can turn it around. Maybe we will. We humans are extremely resourceful. If we could realize we're facing extinction, then my hope is we'd be able to say as a species this is what we have to do. I hope we can get off our butts and get it done.

Do you have any further goals for your diet and exercise program?

Well, a whole food, plant-based, no-oil, starch-based diet is my primary goal. I want to keep eating as cleanly and healthily, and happily, as possible. That means eating at least 90 percent of my meals at home and making things from scratch. I don't even look at all the packaged food in the aisles. The only package I think I get is the bag of rolled oats that I buy. I would say 90 percent of what we eat comes out of the fruit, grain, dried bean, or vegetable bins in the grocery store.

With exercise, I am walking an average of one hour a day with my dog. As my energy improves my goal is to include a fitness class at least three times per week. On YouTube there's Jessica Smith. She is one of my favorite fitness people. It's like the old days in the 80s when we used to do the aerobics classes. I used to love those. I am getting back into that and even in this small room here, I can just shift the table a bit, turn the computer on and get one of her classes going. She does classes for people who only have small spaces for exercise. I am starting with the 10 minute sessions, and then I want to start doing the 20 minute classes, and then 30 minutes and so on. I want to get my fitness to the point where if ever I'm in a situation and I had to run as fast as I could down the street for a couple of blocks, I could do it without collapsing and dying. If we have a tsunami heading our way, I'd like to be able to run a bit.

What about saving the world?

Being part of this group and creating these books is a start. I think that is going to solidify more of what we are talking about, about what needs to be done. In fact, I have often had this quiet voice in me that is saying I've got to write a book about the environment and how it relates to my work doing fertility. How getting to be your fertile best can help the environment, and how that will go on to help the children you're working so hard to have. The idea that your future children will be able to have a future. Just to put that all together and have a little book that people can actually sit down to read and in 100 pages they go, "Alright now, I know what we have to do if we are going to have a chance at slowing down climate change, keep the species going, and give my children and grandchildren a chance to live a full and long life."

What about family relationships? Do you hope for any improvement there?

Oh yes, it's already improved. Since becoming starch-based and avoiding oil, my husband has noticed a big change in my mood. I think eating a lot of potatoes, brown rice, and oatmeal is the main reason for how I feel because you are getting those healthy complex carbohydrates. We know the unrefined carbohydrates are important for secreting serotonin in the brain. Serotonin is a feel-good kind of hormone. If we don't have very much of it we get nasty. I do notice that I am more in love with my husband, and I think that's a big deal after 29 years of marriage.

What do you say to people who would prefer to follow the Paleo diet?

You will probably feel better eating the Paleo diet because you have gotten rid of a lot of junk food and so on. However, I will tell you that the research clearly shows that the Paleo diet will not reverse heart disease. The Paleo diet will not turn diabetes around or arrest cancer or put Lupus, MS or arthritis into remission. Never. The only diet that will make those monumental changes in your health and well-being is a no-oil, whole food, plant-based diet. That is the bottom line. It is the science that supports it. So you have a choice. You can either continue to believe the unscientific nonsense that the Paleo diet is healthy, or you can trust the science and go plant-based.

With a plant-based diet, your sex life is better for both men and women. As a man gets older, erections tend to be not as strong. Sex may still be good but they notice that they don't have as satisfying a time of it as they did when they were younger. When men turn to a whole food plant-based diet, their sex drive goes up and their erections are better. Plus, it is the best diet for long term health, longevity and fertility.

Have you converted anybody to your way of eating?

I suppose I've converted some of my patients. My daughter is a convert, but not due to me, it was due to Gary Yourofsky. I'm hoping as time goes on that my husband will be 100 percent on board. For now, he's at least 90 percent and that's amazing, but 100 percent would be better! I hope this book we're doing will help more people to follow a plant-based diet. Even to do it 80 percent of the time, and allow two to three meals per week with animal foods, if that's still really important to them.

Anything else you'd like to share?

I feel that I'm privileged and so lucky to have found Dr. McDougall and to have learned from him the best way to eat for my health, for the animals, and for the planet. I intend to keep spreading the word, to encourage people who may believe that they're at the end of their rope that there is a way to turn their lives around. I just want to end with saying a really big, heartfelt thank you to Dr. McDougall, and to his wife Mary. They're a great team, and I wish them many more years of success.

Chapter Fifteen
Dom

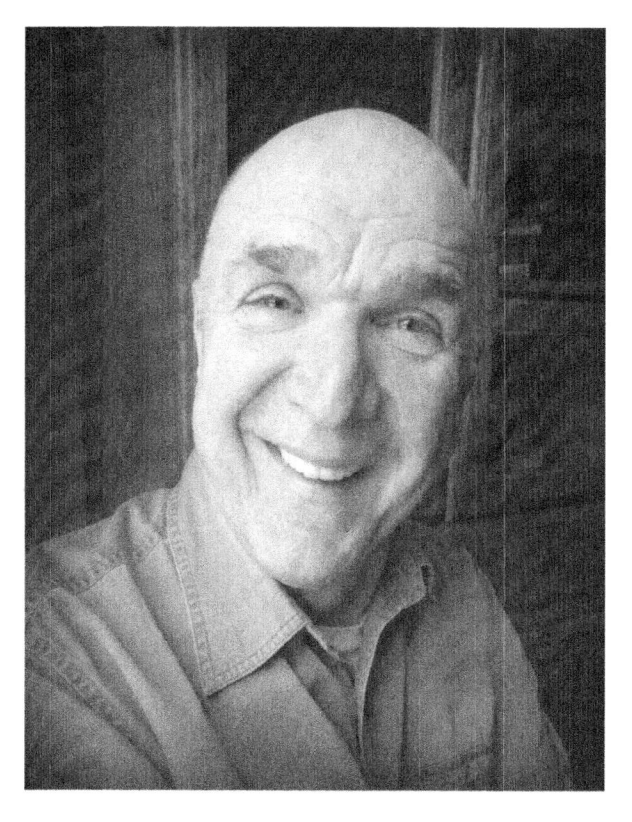

Having lived with a McDougaller for many years, it was easy for Dom to slowly transition to a whole food plant-based diet and reap the extraordinary benefits. His chronic health issues have virtually disappeared, and now, at 63 years of age, he lives pain-free, and takes no medications.

Chapter Fifteen - Dom's Interview

Can you tell us how you came to know Dr. McDougall and his program *The Starch Solution*?

My wife Judith is a McDougaller and she introduced me to him and the philosophy. I have been to the Toronto Starch Solution Meetup group three times. One day I went and enjoyed Dr. McDougall's talk. He was live via Skype and I listened to him speak then. Judith follows him at home so I am sort of indirectly involved with the group. I don't attend the group regularly but I have gotten to know some of the people there. It is very interesting and I do enjoy the food.

How long have you been following this and have you had any health issues that have resolved by following this plant-based, starch-centered diet?

Well, I haven't been doing it as long as Judith. At home, I do participate. I do eat what she eats and we eat together. As far as issues, I had acid reflux problems and I didn't want to take the medications. Judith is a naturopath and told me that I should get off dairy. That was five years ago. She said I would have to be off it for at least three months, not just a week or two, to see if there was a difference. I did it for three months and I didn't have any more problems. I have been completely off all dairy for over five years and I follow it 100 percent. With the acid reflux, I get the occasional flare up but it is very rare. It probably happens when I am sitting on the couch and I let my body sag. That could open the valve on the stomach and I might get acid reflux. If I maintain my posture, then I don't have a problem with it.

Another problem that I had was when Judith and I would go for long walks and I would have severe back pain. I would have to stop and sit every 10 minutes or so. Now, I can go for these long walks and I don't have any more pain. I was also diagnosed with diverticulitis some years ago, but since I've been off dairy and eating mostly plant-based, I don't have any more digestive problems. No more flare ups.

Have you lost any weight?

I don't weigh myself. I just tend to go by how my pants and belt fit. I can just tell. I may have lost four or five pounds but the thing I haven't done, is I haven't eliminated oil. I have reduced my oil intake by 60 percent. I don't use butter, but I would put olive oil everywhere. I'm Italian, and my olive oil is very important to me. I don't know if I could ever completely give it up. I will admit that not putting it everywhere has made a difference as far as feeling lighter. I have always loved starches. I eat a lot of greens and fruits. I exercise. I swim. I burn a lot of starches and carbs.

What about meat?

When I went off dairy, I decided I would be vegan at home, because my daughter always corrects me. She says, "Dad, you're not vegan." I say to her, "You know what I mean." She says, "I know Dad, but you are not vegan." So I go, "Yeah, I am plant-based." I am probably 90 percent plant-based. I do still have a little bit of meat, but not much. I have eliminated chicken from my diet. I think it has been a year now since I've eaten any chicken. I used to do the odd chicken wings with the guys, but now I don't do that anymore. I've found that the smell of chicken is a real turn-off. Honestly, it smells disgusting to me now. I do have a little fish now and then, and I am still a bit of a pork lover. If I am going to eat a bit of meat, I'll have a small amount of pork. Other than that, I don't have much meat at all. It makes up a very small part of my total diet. In a month, I may have meat two or three times, and each time, I eat half of what I used to. My diet has changed a lot and when I tell people my age they go really? I am going to be 64 in November.

Exercise and diet has always been a great big part of my life. Even before I met Judith, being Italian, we ate the so-called Mediterranean diet. I ate a lot of legumes and beans as far back as I can remember. Meat was never a big part of my diet. It was a side dish. It hasn't been a big stretch for me to go meatless at home. When I go out with my friends, they ask me if I don't eat meat, because I am always ordering these vegetable side dishes as my main dish. I think the main reason I don't care to eat meat very often is because it affects my digestion. I feel heavier, and it takes a lot longer for me to digest my meal. I've learned that I can't eat animal foods for dinner if I want to sleep well. Instead, if I'm going to have some fish or pork, I'll eat it for lunch. That gives me at least 10 hours to digest and lets me have a better sleep that night.

In the last five years, since my diet has changed, I feel better. I feel lighter, I have more energy. I still wish I had even more energy. I don't think it has got to do with my diet. Sometimes my B_{12} is low and I take B_{12} supplements. My doctor says everything is fine. It is just that my energy is sometimes low. I would say I generally have more energy since I changed my diet. I think with getting older, we all have less energy.

I disagree. At 64, I am a bit older than you, and I have more energy than I have had in 35 years. It's the oil in your food, Dom. Trust me, the oil you're having is clogging your arteries. Oil makes you lethargic.

I will have to try to get rid of the oil. I have been thinking about it, but when I go out to eat, it's hard to avoid it. There's oil on everything you order in a restaurant. If you have a meal at a friend's house, everything's been cooked in oil. There's even oil in the salad dressings, so eliminating oil is a challenge.

When I'm ready, I'll try to not eat any oil and see if I have more energy. This is my next challenge, to eliminate oil completely from my diet, and see if I do notice the difference in my energy levels and the way I feel. I believe in a slow conversion. I don't believe in doing things cold turkey, but I am open to trying new things and seeing if I feel better.

People say to me, "Dom, don't you miss cheese?" After doing this for five years, I don't think of it anymore but I feel better. If I wouldn't have felt better, I probably would have gone back to cheese, but because I feel better, why go back to something that isn't good for you to begin with?

What kinds of things do you like to eat?

Pasta! Pasta is a favorite. I go in phases. I like to break routines so I have fruit in the morning. If I don't do that then I have my fruits in between my meals. I'll never have fruit after a meal, because I've found that it will give me gas if I do that. Usually in the morning, I'll have a toast or I am a big cookie fan from when I was a kid. I love cookies. I like simple cookies, not chocolate-filled, just a plain biscuit. I am a dunker, so I love dunking cookies in my coffee. Oh boy, if I want to eliminate oil, I'll have to find a fat-free cookie recipe!

I love to eat falafel wraps. That is one of my favorites. I know they are fried so that is now a problem. I'll have to have just the chick peas, not the fried falafel. I know that's why they taste so good, it's all that fatty fried taste. Somebody said you can bake them. Someone else said to me, you can make them half-baked, and half-fried because all baked wouldn't taste as good. I would be willing to try because it is one of my favorite dishes.

Pasta is another favorite dish of mine, but what I do is, I add vegetables to most of my pasta dishes, a lot of veggies. I am a big minestrone lover, so I make soup. I make a minestrone soup at least once a week, and I vary it all the time. I make tomato sauce periodically, but not very often.

Do you cook your sauces from scratch?

Yeah, I chop tomatoes and make a very light tomato sauce with basil. I use canned tomatoes as well. You can make a good sauce by opening a jar of simple tomato sauce. I also like to eat a lot of rice. Judith introduced me to short grain brown rice, and I like it much better than the long grain brown rice. We consume quite a bit of rice, lentils, and beans. I love all of them. I cooked a bunch of white peas in the pressure cooker yesterday. We always have beans in the fridge, all different kinds of beans, all cooked and ready to go, to put into different dishes.

Judith makes hummus with sweet potato and no oil, and I love that.

People ask me what I buy when I go to the market. When I go, I buy lots of greens, fruit and vegetables. You never see me buying meat. I don't buy chicken. You will never see me bring that home because this is a vegan household. When I do eat meat, it is always outside of the house. I eat salads in the summer. I do love salads and I love soups. I like cooked vegetables more often than raw. I love beets. You name the vegetable, and I probably have eaten it.

What about coffee, tea, and alcohol, do you get into that?

I love coffee and I don't have more than two or three small espressos a day. I usually consume them by noon and that's it for the rest of the day. I don't sleep well and that has been a big, big, problem since I was in my 20s. Maybe, it's time to try decaf! I tried it once before when Judith was going to school to become a naturopath. I was seeing a naturopath at the time, and she said you must go off coffee. I said I know it's not the coffee but I will do it. I was off coffee for nine months and there was no difference in my sleep patterns. I drink espresso just because it is short, and has less caffeine. I don't have these tall mugs of coffee that people drink. There is not a lot of caffeine content in espresso. I drink some herbal tea and chicory root coffee as well.

I do love red wine, and the odd beer, but I am not big on spirits. I have a glass of wine at four in the afternoon, but you will rarely see me with a glass of wine past six. The wine would interfere with my sleeping. As we get older, we must make certain adjustments.

Do your friends and family criticize you or question you about eating this way?

Not my family, it is my friends. They say, "Dom, you don't sleep because you don't eat cheese. Dom, you don't sleep because of too much swimming!" What I do is, the people that are savvy, I try to explain it to them, but the people that are hard core, it's just a waste of time. A lot of people out there are just ignorant and to the best of your ability, you can try to explain it to them, but they won't listen. "No, meat is good for you. You've got to eat meat for that protein." I say, "Not really." There are a couple of people I will not broach the subject to, but the ones that are open, then I try to make them aware. However, you are always going to get resistance out there.

With the dairy industry, I get into that sometimes with people because it is a big scam. We are the only species that consumes another animal's milk. We don't need it. No, you don't need the calcium and Judith has taught me that milk and meat leeches the calcium from your bones. You can get calcium in all kinds of other ways like with greens and beans. They're full of calcium. I have those discussions with people. When I go out and they see me eating the way I do, they will say, "Oh, you don't eat meat." I'll answer them, "Yes, I do, but we consume far too much meat." Then, I get into that discussion with them.

What about the stigma that is attached to men about how you are not a real man if you don't eat meat?

I guess I am not a man's man. A lot of guys do think that way. I never did. I always liked my male friends, but I have always enjoyed my women friends' company more than some of the guys. I can't get into that whole male locker room mentality that I was part of when I was in phys-ed. I played a lot of sports. The locker room talk was never my thing. I was a male playing sports but I was doing musical theatre too at the age of 17. I was hanging out with a lot of people that were very effeminate. You can understand the reaction of some of my friends that were jocks because I was considered a jock but not really. They saw me doing all this other stuff and that is why that whole jock thing was never my scene. I never bought into that whole thing, that I'm not a real man if I am not barbecuing every night.

What about your doctor?

The next time I go see him for my check up, I am going to tell him a little bit more about how I've changed my diet. His wife is vegetarian and that is why we touched a little bit on meat because I said I don't consume a lot of meat and if I do it is some pork. He said, "You are not getting B_{12} from pork. You can only get B_{12} from red meat." It turns out my B_{12} is a bit low so I take B_{12} supplements now. Judith had said the same thing, stay on three tablets a week to maintain the B_{12}. I am doing that.

My doctor knows I don't consume a lot of meat and he knows I have been off all cheese for the last five years. He is cool with that. We never really got into you should eat this or that. When I had my last check up, he looked at my triglycerides, and he said, I have unbelievable numbers. He said that I am in the upper 90th percentile, when it comes to triglycerides, and good and bad cholesterol. He says my weight has been pretty well the same for the last 10 years. Yeah, he's got no issues with me eating plant-based. He said I should lose 10 pounds, but other than that, I am in good health.

How are you going to lose the 10 pounds?

Go off the oil! That was a loaded question! I'll probably do that.

When you go to parties and there is this big spread of meat and cheese, what do you do?

In fact, I recently went out to an awards night with my daughter Juliana at a downtown hotel. There were a lot of appetizers being served around the room. Nearly all of them were covered in cheese, seafood, or meat. For example, they had these little sliders, little burgers with cheese, and of course I passed on those. Most people would think, isn't that a great thing to eat? For me, I know they would make me feel ill. It ended up that the only thing I ate was perogies with gravy. Even with that, I had to ask the server to go into the kitchen and find me some perogies without cheese. Juliana, being a vegan, didn't have anything at all. It would be nice to go to a place that is vegan friendly, but that's still not part of our modern world. They cater to the masses. You end up not participating in a lot of what is there. Besides the perogies, I had a beer and that was it.

Do you often take food with you when you go to parties and gatherings with your friends?

I try to eat before I go out. My Dad taught me that. "Eat before you go out." "But Dad, there is going to be food." "Never mind, eat before you go out, because A, it may not be to your liking and B, you might be starving long before the food is served." Back then, when I was growing up, the weddings would start serving dinner at 7 or 8 o'clock and my dad was used to eating at 4:45 in the afternoon. My father didn't like eating that late. We always ate before we went. I remember my uncle would be miserable and wanting to know when the food was coming out because he was so hungry. My father would say, "Ha ha, we've eaten." That always stayed in the back of my mind. Especially today, when you are going to go to an outing and it is a sit-down dinner and they are going to have lots of meat dishes that you can't eat. Eat beforehand, because you are not sure what's going to be on the menu.

Do you carry food in your car?

Yeah, if I know I am doing something, I'll carry food with me. There is nothing worse than getting caught at lunch time when you are starving and there is nothing but fast food restaurants. What I do when I am downtown, I'll go to the vegan restaurant, Fresh. They have a tofu wrap that I love. I will also stop when I am hungry at the falafel place that I like. I seldom stop at a regular restaurant. I haven't gone to fast food restaurants in years.

I guess there are more and more restaurants that are catering to people like you and me now. I am noticing more vegan dishes everywhere. I don't know if it is actually trending, but I think there is a big movement in that direction. I am all for it. It is all about the way you feel. Plant-based food makes you feel better. If everyone would consume 80 percent less of meat and dairy it would be a huge improvement for the environment for many reasons. People say they don't really consume a lot of meat. Really? You had chicken one night, fish the next, pork the next, and then lamb the next, and beef the next, and cheese the next. That is way too much. Then, they stop for burgers three times a week. Just the thought of it, especially with all the obesity we're seeing these days.

What have been your challenges living with a McDougaller?

Well, you know I live with two McDougallers, my daughter and my wife. Judith is more of a McDougaller than my daughter is. Sometimes I forget, and I cook with oil just out of old habits. It calls for a teaspoon of oil, and then Judith won't eat it. I just forget. I am learning to use water instead of the oil, and if I really want the oil I can add a little bit for me on my portion. I am making adjustments. I am not perfect yet. I hit the mark about 80 percent of the time.

Do you feel deprived living with a McDougaller?

No. I am very easy going. If I really want to do something, I'll find a way of doing it somehow. I enjoy eating what my wife and daughter eat. I am not saying, "No! I want my beef! BRING ME BEEF,

WOMAN!" One thing that I admit is, I love bread and to be truthful, I'll bring bread home on the weekend. I'll buy it once a week. I used to bring bread into the house all week long but Judith asked me to stop doing that because it's really hard for her to resist those delicious Italian loaves. Judith tries to avoid bread because she is losing weight. I sometimes like a little bit more salt than she does. She cooks with no salt and I add a little bit if I want, so that is an easy fix.

Do you have any advice for beginners who want to improve their health and start this way of eating?

I would say join the Toronto Starch Solution Meetup group or start your own group if there isn't one where you live. Get involved and meet others who are doing the same thing. I haven't done that personally yet, apart from attending several of those Sunday potlucks. Also, go online and look up Dr. McDougall. I have mentioned him to a couple of people, and have told them to go online and listen to this guy speak, and see if it sparks an interest. I think it is about eating healthy. If you tell people that, then they may want to know exactly what you do and they can go from there. It is easy for me because I was brought into it by Judith and I am getting enough support at home with Juliana and Judith. I don't really need a support group. I do go once in awhile because I really like the food, but it's not like, I must go to the session to be aware of what is going on. Judith keeps me apprised of any changes or new things that come up.

What about the impact of eating whole foods and a vegan diet on the environment and animal rights, do you have any thoughts about that?

Well, my daughter is an ethical vegan and animal activist, and she has made me very aware of that. I hear more than I'd like, actually, to ad nauseam. She is also 22 so I can understand her passion. Yes, thanks to my daughter, I am very aware of the impact of eating animals on the environment. I always remember when we went to Nova Scotia, all four of us, and we stopped at Wolfville to check out the theatre that Christopher Plummer endorsed and had donated money to. When we got there and we got out of the car, there was this stench in the air. I know what farm land smells like because of the manure, but this wasn't manure. I asked a local, what the hell is that smell? Oh that is liquid manure. It is exactly that. They spray the fields with a liquid manure.

How do they extract this liquid manure to spray the plants and the fields?

If you look into things further, you'll hear about these giant hog farms that are so huge that the runoff is liquid. It doesn't have time to sit and break down and do its proper thing because there's just too much of it. I am very aware of these massive farms, and how they are not the way to go. Years ago, people would consume much less meat. They would raise just a couple of animals and that was their food for the year. There was a balance. Right now, I think there is massive consumption and whether it be chickens or hogs or steers, there is too much of it. We are using up a lot of space and a lot of water. The land and water systems cannot handle the load of waste from these giant farms.

That is what Juliana has been teaching me about. I am very much aware. Even in South America I am very aware of what is happening. We keep clearcutting forests, just to make more space to raise cattle, because there is a lot of money in raising cattle. Unfortunately, we are destroying the environment, just to have more and more grazing land for animals. I am very much aware of what we are doing to the environment by consuming and eating a lot of stuff that we shouldn't.

However, my philosophy differs from Judith's and Juliana's because I am not 100 percent vegan. While I am eating 90 percent plant-based, I am not putting down veganism, but my philosophy is that everybody should be eating at least 80 percent plant-based and only a small percent of animal products if they still want to eat those kinds of things. We would be so much further ahead health wise, and environmentally. Maybe one day I will go completely vegan. I am just not there yet.

Do you see yourself changing the world in any way?

I am too old for that. I am too set in my ways. I think that is for the next generation. I think the way I can still have an influence is by educating the people I meet. As an educator, I can spread the truth. I was teaching a grade six class at a local school recently, and we were talking about diets. I was breaking it down for the students. I asked them, what is a vegetarian diet? What is a vegan diet? We talked a little bit about that. We talked about clearcutting to make more space for the cattle farms.

There are some kids who are very, very knowledgeable and are aware of what is happening. I had two passes for $20 each to McDonald's. At school, in this class of grade seven students, I said we are going to have a little draw for these McDonald passes. Five hands went up and they said, "We don't want to participate." I said to them, "Good for you. Now you know why I am giving the tickets away." By not going to McDonald's, they are making a very powerful statement. Based on what we talked about, there are a growing number of young people who are aware. Thanks to the internet, they are learning about our planet, especially regarding climate change. I think it is the younger generation that is going to make a difference, and create a bit of a dent. They have to because they don't have a choice.

With my generation, a lot of them are just stuck in their ways. For instance, my brother says he is not consuming meat. I go, "Oh, so you don't eat meat anymore?" He said, "No, I don't eat as much meat like I used to." That's the thing, people will say they're not eating meat when in fact they're still eating it every day, just a bit less. I wish people with a lot of health problems such as my brother could find a way to cut it out at least 80 percent. Meat is everywhere and it is easy to get it, and people still eat a lot of it. People don't even realize how much meat they're actually consuming, and how harmful it is to their health.

As soon as you start talking to people, and speaking your truth, sharing what you know, you are influencing kids in school, friends or family members, and so on.

I suppose I am changing the world in my own small way. I always believed that you should live by setting an example. I seldom ask my kids to do something. They've seen me shovelling snow. I'll say to my son, "Adrian, if you want to get up and help me shovel you can help me." There is nothing wrong with that. I wouldn't say, "You must help me. You see what I do." When I go out to eat, it is the same thing. My friends see I am eating very differently from everybody else. I'll get one or two people who will notice and will ask. That opens the discussion and I'll have an opportunity to make them aware. That is my approach rather than saying bluntly, you shouldn't be eating that because that is not good for you. It is a little too harsh. Vegans have such a bad name. You just say vegan and everybody's back bristles and their face firms up. You must be really careful how you approach this subject of food.

I went to the periodontist and I mentioned that I live in a vegan household. She makes an announcement in a big loud voice to the whole office, "Hey, he lives in a vegan household." What is that about? However, it wasn't meant to be negative. It turns out some of the other people in the office were vegan too, and she was letting them know that. I thought that was amazing.

The thing is, though, that some vegans are hard core and frankly, just plain unlikeable. I would say to them, try to be more open minded. More and more people are coming around, and they're trying to eat less meat and dairy. It can't happen overnight, unfortunately, but it is happening. Try to practice tolerance of others. Diet is such a huge part of our lives because we do it three times a day. It's important that we learn to share our lives with others whose philosophy is not the same. It becomes problematic if you aren't tolerant of others.

I go along with just about everything in our household, and if there is something I feel very strongly about, I know Judith would support me and do the same for me. I certainly enjoy eating this way. It is really good food, especially at the potlucks. The potluck food is delicious, and a pleasure to eat.

How do you prepare your foods at home?

We do all of our potatoes either boiled or baked. I love mashed potatoes with Mary McDougall's vegetable gravy. We were talking about favorite food before. Potatoes are on my list of favorites. I find them very comforting. Potatoes were my Dad's favourite too. Isn't that something? He'd eat potatoes any which way, even raw. He ate them raw when he was a prisoner in Nazi Germany. Potatoes kept him alive. I guess they couldn't find a pot of water to boil them in. When he was a prisoner of war, he would steal some potatoes in the field, and he'd eat them at night back in the camp in the dark. Boy, that dirty, unwashed potato tasted so good. It kept him alive, dirt and all. It was a real comfort food for him. My son Adrian loves them too. When we make mashed potatoes, I have to ask him if he is going to leave some potatoes for the rest of us.

When I was a kid, we used olive oil. Then, back in the sixties and seventies, there was this huge movement about olive oil being bad for you. Everybody switched to corn oil and that lasted for quite a few years. Then, another study came out and they said corn oil and vegetable oil was bad for you. But olive oil, specifically extra virgin olive oil, was good for you again. It was considered the best oil. That was the trend for the longest time, even to this day, over anything else. Now I'm learning that all oil is bad for us.

A lot of people aren't aware that olive oil is bad. There is such an obesity problem in the world now. It is the oil in everybody's food that is making them fat. Oil is used in all kinds of foods. Look at cookies. Look at the type of oil they are made with, trans fats, the worst kind of fat that clogs your arteries and organs.

I have taken a liking to these crackers called rye crisp thins. They have no oil, but you have to read the labels. Companies put oil, sugar and white flour in just about everything. Gone are the days where you bought without reading the ingredients. Now, you have to read the labels, and you have to know what the synonyms are for some ingredients. They say if you can't pronounce it, it's not good for you. They've got four or five different names for trans fats, but if you don't know what they are, you are still consuming them. The manufacturers shouldn't be allowed to do that, but they are doing it because it's all about the money.

The labelling law that our former prime minister passed federally wasn't as stringent as it should have been, so there are loop holes allowing food companies the opportunity to make a profit at the expense of the general population's health. That is so wrong. This is criminal in my opinion. I should have the right when I buy a product to know exactly what is in it. If I can see what is in it, then I have a choice not to buy it. You want to try and sell me that product with the ingredients disguised under a different name, sneaking that ingredient in there, and I am paying for it and eating it without knowing. That is so wrong.

What these big corporations get away with, it should be criminal. Monsanto is the biggest criminal of all. I have known about them for years, about what they have been doing. It is just awful and yet they keep getting away with it. There is no legislation to rein them in. That is the problem with these corporations, they can commit murder. They do murder people with their unhealthy food ingredients and pharmaceutical drugs, but they are not accountable.

We have been buying organic as early as Adrian was born, which was 28 years ago. We started buying organic in Vancouver. That was such a big part of our budget. We spent a lot of money on organic food. Judith would prepare organic peas and carrots for our babies, by cooking them and making them into a puree, and that is what my kids would eat. We didn't buy jars of baby food. Only the odd one and it was always organic, and that is what we did for years. There are some vegetables we buy that are not organic, if they are not on the dirty dozen list. Otherwise, we don't buy them unless they are organic. If people want to know what's on the list, just google and you'll get all the information.

I think one of the reasons that I am as healthy as I am is because of my consumption of organic food versus all the other food that's out there. That has probably saved my life. Look at me, for somebody who is 63, I have never had any surgeries. I have never been on any medications. I don't even take aspirin. I don't take any painkillers. I see people popping Advil all the time. I never use any of that stuff. I am very lucky in that respect, but no, it is not luck, it is the food! I eat well and that makes a difference.

In fact, I talked to a doctor friend who I visit with when I go to the St. Lawrence Market every Saturday. His name is Bill, he's a great guy. He brought it up. I don't pepper him with medical questions. We talk about everything. We talk about theatre. He is a very intelligent man. One day, we touched upon colonoscopies. I have had two. He said he has never had one. He finds it too invasive. He said that unless you have a history in your family, or reason to believe that you are at risk, don't have one.

That got me thinking. I was scheduled for a colonoscopy in a few weeks and they kept calling, and I said I am going to be talking to my doctor but I am not going to have one. It's because my diet is what it is, I don't feel that I need one. I am going to pass on it and my doctor can't force me to have one. Even Judith said, "Dom, it is very invasive. There is no reason why you should have it. You poop at least twice a day."

Since then, I've learned that for the number of people that they save by finding a cancer polyp, they kill the same number of other people doing the procedure. It is a wash statistically. It doesn't happen often but a perforation can occur. So, now I have decided, I am not going to have it anymore. I am going to go for a physical, but I am passing on the colonoscopy. I am consuming so little meat and eating so many fruits, vegetables, and healthy starches, I am definitely not at risk for getting colon cancer.

Chapter Sixteen
Murray

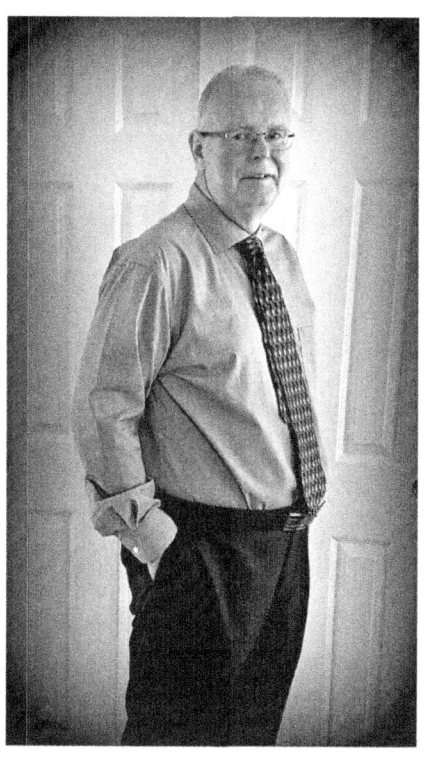

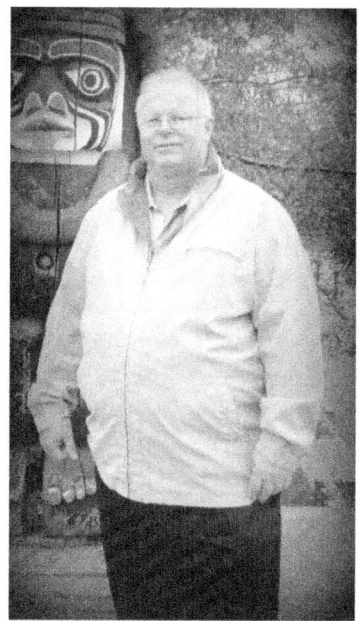

This remarkable story is about a man who has struggled with his health and weight his entire adult life. Murray has tried many diets including the Bernstein diet, the Atkins diet, the Mediterranean diet, and the Paleo diet. None of them ever worked. Then Murray found Dr. McDougall and his revolutionary starch-centered program. Follow Murray on his journey back to health with a weight loss of over 100 pounds.

Toronto Starch Solution Meetup Group
Group Toronto Starch Solution Meetup

Chapter Sixteen - Murray's Interview

Let's start with a bit of back information about you and your life.

Dad was Scottish. Mom was Irish. I come from a small rural farming community in southwest Ontario. My dad owned a construction company. Mom was a stay-at-home mom. I was raised on meat and potatoes, a small portion of vegetables, and then dessert twice a day. We had lots of physical activity. I played sports every day when I was in my teens. I played hockey seven days a week. Then, I went to college and got a degree in business administration with a major in data processing. From there, life got sedentary. I started sitting behind a desk 12 to 14 hours a day. That made a big difference, and I didn't keep up any of the activity. I have one brother. He is extremely heavy. Cancer runs in the family - bowel cancer in particular. I was quite heavy when I started this journey on Dr. McDougall's program. To date, I have lost 93 pounds.

I've got to give you a high five for that. That is awesome!

I've got another 30 pounds to go.

You are doing so well.

I have been doing this for over a year now; that is really not very long. One or two pounds per week of weight loss is what I am trying for. Some months it works, some months it doesn't. When I started, I was 308 pounds. I am 5 feet, 9 inches tall. I was getting to the point where I had a hard time walking around the block. Lori got me started on this. We had several false starts with a number of different types of programs. I think I have been on every diet in the world. I've done everything: Bernstein's diet, the Akins diet, the Mediterranean diet, the Paleo diet. You name it, I have tried it. It was just the yo-yo effect on those ones. First, you'd lose 10-20 pounds and you'd come off it and put the weight back on again. I really needed to do something different. I got to a point a little over a year ago where I said I had to do something and it needed to be more of a lifestyle change than changing my eating habits for a short period of time. Lori and I started experimenting and we found Dr. McDougall's *The Starch Solution* program.

It works well for me, mainly because it is simple. I had psoriasis. I had diabetes. I had high cholesterol. I had a slow thyroid. I had a lot of extra weight - all the diseases of modern man. I think it was from eating all the synthetic, processed foods, quite frankly. I was on 11 or 12 different pills. I am now down to three, plus a small insulin injection.

A by-product of this whole process from eating starch is my psoriasis cleared up. I have had psoriasis since I was 14 years old, and it is gone. It is amazing from that perspective. That is the proof in the pudding that this works. I have energy to spare. Quite frankly, I can walk all the time. Active things are totally different. I feel so much better and healthier. In fact, one of my buddies who hadn't seen me for almost a year said to me, "Man, your skin looks good." He hadn't seen me in a year and I had lost a ton of weight. I have lost it slowly, so I don't have a lot of saggy skin. I think I look healthy.

You look great.

We tried some of the other doctors too, like Dr. Fuhrman, and the *Forks over Knives* program. They were plant-based as well and we mixed and matched. Finally, we arrived at Dr. McDougall's program. I think it has been very good for me. The thing that worked for me is that it is simple. It's easy to do. Half starch, half green vegetables, on my plate works well for me. That is easy to do. It was, however, quite a transition for me. I'll be honest. I'm not perfect by any stretch of the imagination, mainly because of life pressures and peer pressures.

Quite frankly, I like meat. I like the taste of meat. I like the texture. I am always on Lori about the texture of the food. I guess I miss the chewing aspect of meat. I generally stick pretty close to the program now. I probably have one to two meals a week where I am not in sync with the program, and probably more, when I am travelling. The last two weeks have been tough. I have been on four business trips in two weeks, New York, Miami, New Jersey, and Edmonton. Living in hotels and eating in restaurants, it becomes extremely difficult to stay on the program. Even if you ask for something simple, there is always something oily on it. Oil is everywhere. It really is.

Is your cholesterol way down then?

My health has improved quite a bit. Here is a list of all the drugs I am off: I dropped one pill for blood pressure, one pill for acid reflux, two pills for cholesterol, one pill for diabetes, two insulin injections for diabetes, one injection for psoriasis, and a water pill. I stopped taking aspirin. I have dropped all of these. I only have one blood pressure pill, one thyroid pill, and one cholesterol pill left, and a daily shot of insulin for diabetes. Ideally, I'd like to get off everything I can, and that is what I am driving towards.

I am hoping to get off that last cholesterol medicine shortly. My cholesterol was normal the last time I saw the doctor. He took me off one pill and left me on two, and I took myself off one. I am seeing him in another two months. I am still taking a thyroid pill, which is a different class of drugs, but I still take it. Essentially, I have come off of nine pills in total so far.

I go to a heart and kidney specialist. My blood specialist recommended me to him because I had some protein in my urine. I go see him every six months now. He is amazed with what is happening to me. It's the same with my diabetic doctor. I told him I am leaving my blood sugar a little high because insulin slows down the weight loss, and my goal is to lose all this weight. I have had my challenges. I have hit a lot of plateaus.

When I first met you, you were on a plateau.

I dropped a few pounds since then, and now I am on a plateau again. The way I look at it is there are only three things that cause weight gain. It is hereditary, it is what you eat, or it is about the exercise. In the summertime, it is not hard to get some exercise regularly with the pool, treadmill, and golf. Winter time is a little harder. I have the treadmill downstairs. The challenge is to be disciplined enough to do 30 minutes to an hour every day and keep my activity up.

How did you discover Dr. McDougall?

Lori hit me across the back of the head with this and said, "You are going to do this". She has converted me.

What are the kinds of things you like to eat?

I have porridge every morning with berries. I take a banana to work. I have only two fruits a day. Typically, I take rice or potatoes for lunch, with celery and carrots to eat in the office. I like it simple. I like rice. I like beans. I like potatoes. I like salads. That is primarily what we eat.

It's great when you understand how tasty simple food is. You don't have to cook like crazy.

For me, the journey has been good, with lots of trials and tribulations. I went to a golf course today. I had a tomato sandwich and a fruit bowl. The boys had sausages, hot dogs, and sweet potato fries. I am eating differently and I have lots of peer pressure. Sometimes, you see people roll their eyes when you ask them to do something special at a restaurant.

As you know, the McDougall people are in the minority. There are lots of vegans and there are lots of vegetarians, but the concept of a no oil diet is extreme for most. It's so important in our current food environment to understand about oil. McDougall and his whole concept of not having oil is critical to getting your health back. Cleaning out your cells of fat solves so many health problems for us. I believe that's why my psoriasis disappeared. Unclogged cells will reverse diabetes and clean out arteries of the fat sludge that's accumulated, and all those types of things.

My biggest challenges have been plateaus. I follow the program faithfully but at times I am just stuck. I just love to eat. I was raised that way. Plateaus are the one thing I fight all the time. How I look - self-awareness. My co-workers have really supported me. My friends have really supported me. They understand. If I am going to have a cheat meal, it is typically with them because it is easier and less confrontational.

My doctors are all on board about this. There is no doubt about that. My heart and kidney specialist, my endocrinologist, and my family doctor are all on board with it and they are all amazed. My family doctor at one point was talking to me about having a gastric by-pass because I couldn't lose this weight. I didn't see him for about eight months on purpose and then went in. He didn't recognize me. He had to take a second and third look. It was amazing.

I like your route way better than his route. Where is your support coming from?

It is Lori. She is in the house right now cooking dinner for us.

Who else has influenced you? Were you on YouTube soaking up all that healthy information from all those other great hero doctors?

You know, I have not done any of that. The only thing I do is read, or watch the clips that Lori sends to me. If she sends me a video to watch on whatever subject, I watch it. For example, she'll go through a McDougall video and say, "Watch the first five minutes, watch from 20-23 minutes, and watch the last five minutes." That is what I do.

Do you have any advice for beginners?

Yes, keep it simple. When I started this, Lori hadn't moved back in yet so I was living as a single person. I hated cooking for myself. Cooking for two is easy, but cooking for myself was a challenge. I wasn't going to put together complex meals. We have a beginner in our family. My daughter has not lost the weight she gained from her pregnancies. She is having a real problem so we introduced her to Dr. McDougall's program. She is trying it and she has been doing it for over two and a half weeks and has lost 10 pounds so far.

You must be so thrilled that she is on it!

Yes, of course, I'm really glad she's giving it a try. As far as advice for beginners, I think it's best to just keep it simple. Have lots of simple types of sauces for your rice and beans whether it is hot sauce or Thai sauce or a variety so you are changing it up all the time. That is what keeps you from getting bored. The foundation is simple: rice, beans and potatoes. Then, add vegetables and fruit to that.

Do you make your own sauces or do you buy prepared sauces?

Lori makes our salad dressings and gravy. We buy everything else.

What can you do now that you couldn't do a year ago?

From a mental perspective, I am much more aware of what I eat. I can tell when there is oil on stuff and I won't eat fried foods. I used to love takeout fried chicken. About six months ago, I tried a piece. I bought a two-piece snack pack and I couldn't eat it. I had one bite and I couldn't stand the taste of the oil. Dr. McDougall and Dr. Fuhrman did advise us that our tastes will change as we embrace this new way of eating and we would grow to like the food. My tastes have changed substantially to where I really don't want anything greasy or with fat on it. It doesn't taste good to me.

What I can do now that I couldn't do a year ago is my activity level is better. I'm not tired like I used to be. In the past, when I got home from work, I would eat sitting on the couch for an hour, and then go to bed. Now I'm up until 10 or 11 with lots more energy. I am happy to walk around the block. I have a newfound activity level that feels great. I suspect Lori would tell you that I am not quite as moody as I use to be. It is all positive, quite frankly.

When you think about it, food must have some effect on brain chemistry.

It must have. I think that was a big part of the problem with eating meat and vegetables, or eating meat and salad, or meat without any starch. Anything that I have ever learned about dieting in the past was it was always low carb, low carb, low carb. This McDougall program is the reverse. When you think about it, our systems, our muscles and our brains all run on glycogen, which is made from carbohydrates. No wonder we are moody if we are not eating the fuel that our brains and body require to function properly.

A lot has been said about the impact of a whole food, plant-based

diet on the environment and animal rights. What are your thoughts on that?

In my opinion, each to their own, quite frankly. I was raised in a small farming community. I worked in a butcher shop. I used to hunt. From my perspective, if animals are hunted or raised ethically, and used completely, that is acceptable. Most animals have been raised for that purpose. But, it is a personal choice what you want to eat. There is just way too much commercialization on both the animal side and the whole plant food side of it.

For example, let's look at the gluten thing. Marketing and advertising, everything has gluten-free on it. Whatever the buzz words are, they are going to try to market it and sell it. People should have the freedom to live the life they want. They should be able to live in a manner they want to, that is going to be able to provide the health level they are looking for. There are people who can eat meat and potatoes, and don't have any health problems, depending on their hereditary factors. And, there are people like myself who can't eat meat anymore. You have to come to those realizations yourself. Everybody is different. Everybody is an individual. The food you put in your body is the number one, most important thing that affects your health.

What are your future goals related to health and weight loss?

To lose 30 more pounds!

Thirty more pounds, you are already three quarters of the way there. That is fantastic!

When you look at the BMI scales it doesn't take into consideration your muscle mass. They try to peg everybody into one type of chart. I don't believe it is accurate. I believe that body mass is comprised of bone structure, and muscle density as well as fat. When I get down to 195 pounds, which is where I want to be, that will be the perfect weight for me. I am at 213 pounds right now.

That is so great. You must feel fantastic!

I do. The best part of the McDougall program is that it is a lifestyle. As long as you follow it, the weight is not going to come back on. It is an easy and a tasty lifestyle to follow. That is the other great part.

Is this for the rest of your life?

Yup. I go up and down two or three pounds but it is like it never gets away from you. I know the lifestyle I must follow to stay thin and healthy now.

Do you see yourself changing the world in any way?

I don't. I don't see myself changing the world. I see myself changing myself and helping my family. If I can look after myself and look after my family, and keep them healthy and live within the structures of the world, I think that is all I can do.

Have you converted anybody to this way of eating?

Well, we think we have converted our daughter. I have had a lot of people ask me about it. I don't push it on them. When they ask, I just say this is what is working for me. Here, look up Dr. McDougall on YouTube, and listen to him. If you are interested, try it. If you don't, that is your own personal choice, and we go from there.

Do you think there is a chance they could change some laws around food and drugs?

I think it is a long, long way out there. Organics have been around forever and then you had to become certified to become organic, so the government is involved again to regulate it. Now, it is totally commercialized.

Don't you think it is good thing that the government is regulating it? People can't say it's organic when it's not. It's good to have standards.

I understand that, but now it becomes a marketing scenario. It's organic, so now it is twice as expensive. Organic vegetables should be as affordable as normal vegetables, because the normal vegetables are probably costing more to produce with all the chemicals dumped on them than organic vegetables. I come from a farming community. I know the amount of crap that is put on everything. From a pesticide perspective, the pesticides are not cheap. Why is organic food so much more expensive than regular food? Perhaps, in 10 years, there won't be a pesticide-laced version of vegetables for sale. It won't exist because the market dictates what they produce. It will all be organic because that is what everybody wants and hopefully the price will go back down. The world will change one person at a time. You are making a choice about what vegetables you will buy. If there are 100,000 people making that same choice, then that's what is going to drive the market down.

Humans are herd animals. They follow the largest group of people and they follow the path of least resistance, except for the 5 to 10 percent that want to swim up the stream, and eat healthily, instead of swim down. It is a challenge to be part of the large group, but still be individualistic in the way you are trying to eat. That becomes difficult, and people give up on it because it is too hard. How do you make eating healthy more acceptable from a peer perspective and a society perspective? Those are the things that I think influence people. It is easy to eat healthy if I am sitting at home and following this exactly. If I am travelling two to three weeks out of a month, it is virtually impossible to follow.

It is hard to find greens. It is virtually impossible to find plain rice. It is impossible to find something to eat in the mornings, except porridge, and you are paying 12 dollars for. It becomes extremely difficult when you are travelling and you are on this plan.

I call myself a "flexitarian", not a vegan, because I am flexible. I probably have a bad meal once or twice a week. I do not torture myself when I go out. I don't need the stress. I will try and look for something that is healthy, and most times, it is virtually impossible, but I am getting better at it.

You have grandchildren. They say that the fish are going to be gone out of the ocean in 50 years. Are you worried about that or do you have an opinion about what we can do as humanity as a whole?

I am very worried about natural resources from a food perspective, because we are either polluting fish with too much mercury or we are raising them as farm-raised fish where they are being given antibiotics and pellets to eat. To fix the declining numbers of fish in our oceans, you would have to put a moratorium on all fishing for about 10 to 15 years to bring the stocks back up. I do not see the governments ever doing that because you have all the Newfoundland people, and people from around the world living off fishing and whaling. If you take their livelihood away, you'd have to subsidize their income, and then the tax payer has a burden. Then it becomes a vicious cycle. I don't know where it begins and where it stops. I don't know how to fix it unless you fix it in your own little community by making changes yourself. The answer is very simple, just stop eating fish. Everybody has to stop eating fish.

Let's go back to your doctor for a minute. Did you tell him you were going to try this diet for weight loss?

I didn't tell him. I just did it. I told him that this is the way I am going to stop all these pills and stop this insulin and that is the way it is going to be. I am not asking anybody for anything. I am not asking for permission to do anything.

What about when he saw your results, was he curious at all with what you were doing?

Yes, especially my heart and kidney specialist. He wanted to know exactly everything I was doing. I referred him to *The Starch Solution* and Dr. McDougall, so he could find out what I was doing. I told him what I was doing when I stopped the drugs. He said, "You are doing fabulous." He was totally amazed. He told me that I had been headed for a heart attack and kidney failure. He said that I have reversed everything. He is very pleased for me and extremely supportive.

I think a doctor who follows the medical association rules and what they have been taught as a typical family doctor, is not qualified to give nutritional advice. They only get a few hours of nutritional education in their entire medical training. He can recommend the drug and I can choose to buy it or not buy it, but he is giving that prescription so he is totally covered from a liability perspective. That is where most doctors are today. They all start medical school with good intentions, because they want to help people. Eventually, it becomes how many patients can I see, and how much money can I make.

They don't see anybody getting well because they are treating the symptoms and not the cause of the illness. I think Dr. McDougall's food plan gets right at the root of the problem. It is changing the food which is causing the illness, versus just treating the symptoms. I don't see mainstream doctors following Dr. McDougall because of the liability issue.

I just thought they weren't interested in a nutritional approach because they can't make any money from recommending a diet as opposed to doing a $150,000 bypass surgery.

Lori and I used to go to a doctor who was a naturopath but a medical physician too. He would do half and half. He got sideways with the medical association and instead of going to court, he retired. It was the same type of scenario. A patient complained that he was given naturopathic stuff instead of prescription, and the Medical Association came down on him, so he retired. It wasn't worth the battle. That is the challenge. The medical association, the government, the food association, are all dictating what their professions have to do and what rules they have to follow.

Do you have any desire to go meet Dr. McDougall?

I think it would be interesting to see Dr. McDougall and listen to him. I find the talks on YouTube that Lori tells me to listen to are informative. His desire to cure one person at a time is commendable. I think he is very tired of the same battle he's had repeatedly with Big Food and Big Business. I think he is extremely frustrated over the whole scenario. He knows he could help even more people, but he can't make it happen.

When you stop, and look at it, people call themselves vegan, but look at the amount of oil they have on their food. It's the oil that is hurting them. Some people call themselves vegetarian and they are eating fish and cheese. The labels of the different types of eating are so blurred. I am a vegan, but to go that next step of removing all the refined foods and oils is very difficult for people. You enrol people, one person at a time. If anybody asks me, I tell them what I am doing, but they think it is extreme. I think this is an uphill challenge getting people to try it. I know that in my busy life I will never be that evangelistic type of person. It is just not in me. I am not going to jump up on a stand and tell the world.

I think what happens for most of us is that we get really sick and

then we start looking for a solution, and we are forced to change. Lucky for us, we found the solution, with a whole food, starch-centered, no-oil diet.

I just got to the point where I did not feel good at all, in any part of my day. I knew if I didn't change something, I knew I would die. Now, I am going to see my grandchildren grow up. I just knew I had to do something. Lori came across all these different diets and it started with the movie, *Forks over Knives*. The McDougall plan is the one that stuck and it is working for me. I have lost 93 pounds and counting. It works for a lot of people. I am off nine drugs. The one that I didn't expect is the psoriasis clearing up, and I have had it since puberty. It is finally gone. I haven't needed to take anything for it for nine months now. It is 99 percent gone. I only have one small spot left. It is there to remind me of how far I have come.

Dr. Doug Lisle advocates that if you follow the McDougall program 80 percent of the time, you will lose the weight. You said you are taking your weekends to be a "flexitarian" and it is working for you?

I have gone down from a size 54 pant to a size 40 pant. I am going to be in a 38 shortly. I wasn't even in 38s when I was 17 years old. It is a remarkable change and I am really pleased.

There is a positive sub-text to all of this because you have made this your default lifestyle choice, so your weight gain will never be out of control ever again. You know exactly how you have to eat to maintain it. It has become a lifestyle of choice. Once you get a taste of health again, there is no going back.

I may fall off the wagon on occasion but I am going to climb back on because I know this starch-based, no-added-oil program works and it stabilizes things. Ultimately over time, you come back to the optimal weight that your body wants to be. Nature takes its course.

When I met you the first time in June, you were so frustrated because you had been plateauing. I talked to you about the book, *McDougall's Program for Maximum Weight Loss*. Did you try it so you could get over that hump?

That is what we are doing now. It's slowed down a lot, but I am losing more weight.

Did you ever imagine in your wildest dreams that you could get thin and well again?

No! I never thought I could do this. The other thing is not taking the medications anymore. I feel so much better because I don't have to deal with all the nasty side effects of those drugs. It is a win-win scenario. Thin body, and good health. It really is fantastic. I am much more mellow and happy with life, to be quite honest.

A Last Word

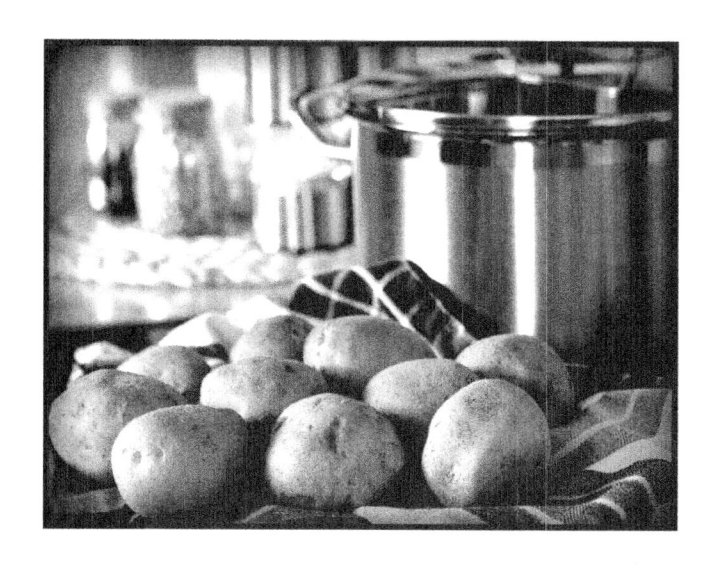

You can do it too.

Toronto Starch Solution Meetup Group

A Last Word from Diane McConnell

You Can Do It Too

Are you tired of being fat and sick? Now you are at that choice point. You are at a cross roads. You have read our incredible success stores. You can make a proactive decision right here, right now, to save your own life. You can circumvent our traditional medical system and take charge of your own well-being. You can take back control of your own health, strength, vitality, and body size. You now understand the healing and destructive power of the food you are putting in your mouth, morning, noon, and night.

You are the one who controls the food that goes in your body. You can choose to eat a whole food, starch-based diet while eliminating the animal products and oil, and allow your body to heal itself. Or, you can continue to eat those poisonous foods of meat, dairy and oil and get sicker and heavier. In no time, you end up taking all sorts of pharmaceutical drugs to try to manage your life-threatening conditions. The solution is simple. It is the food. It has been proven with science and the facts are published in the latest medical journals, that a whole food, low-oil, starch-based diet will heal your body. The solution is low-cost and right at your fingertips.

It is our hope that our stories will inspire you to make the decision to allow your body to heal with a whole food starch-based diet. With this decision, you are not only helping yourself but you are reducing the suffering of the animals, contributing to the healing of our planet's ecosystems, and reducing climate change with no added effort. We wish you all the best in regaining your health and optimal weight.

May the "McDougall McForce" be with you.

All the best,

Diane McConnell

References

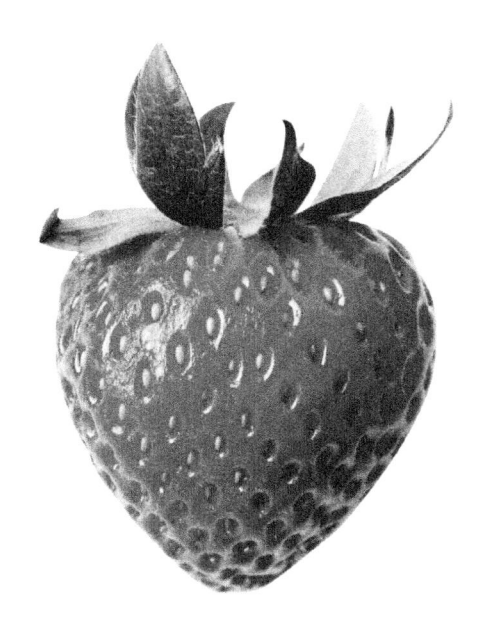

Toronto Starch Solution Meetup Group

References

Chapter One

1) Ng M, Flemin T, Robinson M, Thomson B, Graetz N, et al. Global, regional, and national prevalence of overweight and obesity in children and adults during 1980-2013: a systematic analysis for the Global Burden of Disease Study 2013. *The Lancet*, Vol 384, No 9945, p766-781, Aug 30, 2014.

2) The GBD 2015 Obesity Collaborators, Health Effects of Overweight and Obesity in 195 Countries over 25 Years. *The New England Journal of Medicine*. June 12, 2017. DOI:10.1056/NEJMoa1614362.

3) Benjamin EJ, Blaha MJ, Chiuve SE, Cushman M, Das SR, Deo R, de Ferranti SD, Floyd J, Fornage M, Gillespie C, Isasi CR, Jimenez MC, Jordan LC, Judd SE, Lackland D, Lichtman JH, Lisabeth L, Liu S, Longenecker CT, Mackey RH, Matsushita K, Mozaffarian D, Mussolino ME, Nasir K, Neumar RW, Palaniappan L, Pandey DK, Thiagarajan RR, Reeves MJ, Ritchey M, Rodriguez CJ, Roth GA, Rosamond WD, Sasson C, Towfighi A, Tsao CW, Turner MB, Virani SS, Voeks JH, Willey JZ, Wilkins JT, Wu JHY, Alger HM, Wong SS, Muntner P; on behalf of the American Heart Association Statistics Committee and Stroke Statistics Subcommittee. Heart disease and stroke statistics—2017 update: a report from the American Heart Association [published online ahead of print January 25, 2017]. Circulation. doi: 10.1161/CIR.0000000000000485

4) WHO Mortality Database [online database]. Geneva: World Health Organization; (http://apps.who.int/healthinfo/statistics/mortality/causeofdeath-query/, accessed 12 January 2016).

5) Thorogood M, Mann J, Appleby P, McPherson K. Risk of death from cancer and ischaemic heart disease in meat and non-meat eaters. *Br Med J*. 1994;308:1667-1670.

6) Chang-Claude J, Frentzel-Beyme R, Eilber U. Mortality patterns of German vegetarians after 11 years of follow-up. *Epidemiology*. 1992;3:395-401.

7) Chang-Claude J, Frentzel-Beyme R. Dietary and lifestyle determinants of mortality among German vegetarians. *Int J Epidemiol*. 1993;22:228-236.

8) Fraser GE. Vegetarian diets: what do we know of their effects on common chronic diseases? *Am J Clin Nutr*. 2009 May; 89(5):167S-1612S.

9) Sinha R, Cross AJ, Graubard BI, Leitzmann MF, Schatzkin A. Meat intake and mortality: a prospective study of over half a million people. *Arch Intern Med*. 2009 Mar 23; 169(6):562-71.

10) Subramanian S, Chait A. The effect of dietary cholesterol on macrophage accumulation in adipose tissue: implications for systemic inflammation and atherosclerosis. *Curr Opin Lipidol*. 2009 Feb;20(1):39-44.

11) Morin RJ, Hu B, Peng SK, Sevanian A. Cholesterol oxides and carcinogenesis. *J Clin Lab Anal*. 1991;5(3):219-25.

12) Frassetto L. Diet, evolution and aging--the pathophysiologic effects of the post-agricultural inversion of the potassium-to-sodium and base-to-chloride ratios in the human diet. Eur J Nutr. 2001 Oct;40(5):200-13.

13) McDougall JA, McDougall MA. *The Starch Solution; Eat the foods you love, regain your health, and lose the weight for good!* New York, NY: Rodale, 2012. Print.

14) Adams KM, Butsch WS, Kohlmeier M. The state of nutrition education at US medical schools. *Journal of Biomedical Education*. 2015, Article ID 357627, 7 pages http://dx.doi.org/1.1155/215/357627.

15) Willett WC. Balancing lifestyle and genomics research for disease prevention. *Science*. 202;296(558):695-8.

16) Olshansky SJ, Passaro DJ, Hershow RC, et al. A potential decline in life expectancy in the United States in the 21st century. *N Engl J Med*. 2005;352(11): 1138-45.

17) Wilson GT, in Fairbanks and Wilson (Eds) Binge Eating: Nature, Assessment and Treatment. Guilford Press, New York, NY, 1993. (Wilson cites the work of Bemis "Phobia, Obsession or Addition: What Underlies Eating Disorders?" a paper presented at the National Conference on Eating Disorders, Columbus, Ohio, 1985; Roden and Reed, "Sweetness and Eating Disorders," in Dobbing (Ed) Sweetness; Springer-Verlag, and Wardle "Compulsive Eating and Dietary Restraints," British Journal of Clinical Psychology, 1987).

18) Colantuoni C, et al. "Evidence That Intermittent Excessive Sugar Intake Causes Endogenous Opioid Dependence," *Obesity Research*, 2002. Bernard, op cit, summarizes in lay language that food "contains chemical compounds no one ever suspected were there – mild opiates that are released during digestion. Other researchers have added evidence that there is really something about sugar, chocolate, cheese and meat and certain other foods that set them apart. They don't just tickle the taste buds. It appears they actually stimulate the brain in such a way that it is easy to get hooked and tough to break free, even if you find yourself gaining weight or lapsing into other health problems."

19) Drewnowski A, et al. "Taste Response and Preferences for Sweet High-fat Foods: evidence of opioid involvement," Physical Behavior, 51: p371-9, 1992.

20) Lisle DJ, Goldhamer A. *The Pleasure Trap; Mastering the hidden force that undermines health and happiness*. Summertown, Tenessee: Healthy Living Publications, 2003. Print.

21) Jenkins DJ, Kendall CW, Marchie A, et al. The Garden of Eden – plant based diets, the genetic drive to conserve cholesterol and its im-

plication for heart disease in the 21st century. *Comp Biochem Physiol*, Part A Mol Integr Physiol. 2003;136(1): 141-51.

22) Ornish D, Scherwitz LW, Billings JH, et al. Intensive lifestyle changes for reversal of coronary heart disease. Five-year follow-up of the Lifestyle Heart Trial. *JAMA*. 1998;280(23):2001-7.

23) Kantor ED, Rehm CD, Haas JS, et al. Trends in prescription drug use among adults in the United States from 1999-2012. *JAMA*. 2015; 314(17):1818-1830.

Chapter Three

1) Fraser GE. Vegetarian diets: what do we know of their effects on common chronic diseases? *Am J Clin Nutr*. May 2009; 89(5):167S-1612S.

2) Estes EH, Kerivan L. An archaeologic dig: a rice-fruit diet reverses ECG changes in hypertension. *J Electrocardiol*. Sep. 2009; Vol. 47(5): 599–607.

3) Kapadia CR. Vitamin B_{12} in health and disease: part 1 – inherited disorders of function, absorption, and transport. *Gastroenterologist*. Dec 1995;3(4):329-44.

4) McDougall JA. A starch-based diet supports spontaneous healing. *The McDougall Newsletter*. May 2009, Vol. 8, Issue 5.

5) McDougall JA, McDougall MA. *The Starch Solution; Eat the foods you love, regain your health, and lose the weight for good!* New York, NY: Rodale, 2012. Print.

6) Gomez-Pinilla F, Nguyen TTJ. Natural mood foods: the actions of polyphenols against psychiatric and cognitive disorders. *Nutr Neurosci*. 2012;15(3):127-33.

7) Rooney C., McKinley M.C., Woodside J.V. The potential role of fruit and vegetables in aspects of psychological well-being: A review of the literature and future directions. *Proc. Nutr. Soc.* 2013;72:420–432.

8) White BA, Horwath CC, Conner TS. Many apples a day keep the

blues away – daily experiences of negative and positive affect and food consumption in young adults. *Br J Health Psychol.* 1997;23:94-102.

9) Anderson GH, Woodend D. Effect of glycemic carbohydrates on short-term satiety and food intake. *Nutr Rev.* 2003 May;61(5 Pt 2):S17-26.

10) Bolton-Smith C, Woodward M. Dietary composition and fat to sugar ratios in relation to obesity. Int J Obes Relat Metab Disord. 1994 Dec;18(12):820-8.

11) Poppitt SD, Keogh GF, Prentice AM, Williams DE, Sonnemans HM, Valk EE, Robinson E, Wareham NJ. Long-term effects of ad libitum low-fat, high-carbohydrate diets on body weight and serum lipids in overweight subjects with metabolic syndrome. *Am J Clin Nutr.* 2002 Jan;75(1):11-20.

12) McDougall JA. The fat vegan. *The McDougall Newsletter.* December 2008; Vol. 7, No. 12.

13) McDougall JA. People Passionate about starches are healthy and beautiful. *The McDougall Newsletter.* March 2009, Vol. 8, No. 3.

14) Blundell JE, Lawton CL, Cotton JR, Macdiarmid JI. Control of human appetite: implications for the intake of dietary fat. *Annu Rev Nutr.* 1996;16:285-319.

15) Rolls BJ, Kim-Harris S, Fischman MW, Foltin RW, Moran TH, Stoner SA. Satiety after preloads with different amounts of fat and carbohydrate: implications for obesity. *Am J Clin Nutr.* 1994 Oct;60(4):476-87. *Annu Rev Nutr.* 1996;16:285-319.

16) McDougall JA. Acne has nothing to do with diet – wrong! *The McDougall Newsletter.* Nov 2003; Vol. 2, No. 11.

17) Cordain L. Acne vulgaris: a disease of Western civilization. *Arch Dermatol.* 2002 Dec;138(12):1584-90.

18) Magee EA. Contribution of dietary protein to sulfide production in the large intestine: an in vitro and a controlled feeding study in humans. *Am J Clin Nutr.* 2000 Dec;72(6):1488-94.

19) McDougall JA. Protein Overload. *The McDougall Newsletter*. January 2004, Vol. 3, No. 1.

20) McDougall JA. Five major poisons inherently found in animal foods. *The McDougall Newsletter*. Jan 2010, Vol. 9, Issue 1.

21) Pan A, Sun Q, Bernstein AM, Schulze MB, Manson JE, Stampfer MJ, Willett WC, Hu FB. Red Meat Consumption and Mortality: Results From 2 Prospective Cohort Studies. *Arch Intern Med*. 2012 Mar 12.

22) Hellerstein MK, Schwarz JM, Neese RA. Regulation of hepatic de novo lipogenesis in humans. *Annu Rev Nutr*. 1996;16:523-57.

23) Kon S. XXXV. The value of whole potato in human nutrition. *Biochemical J*. 1928; 2:258-260.

24) Lopez de Romana G. Fasting and postprandial plasma free amino acids of infants and children consuming exclusively potato protein. *J Nutr*. 1981 Oct;111(10): 1766-71.

25) Danforth E Jr. Det and obesity. *Am J Clin Nutr*. 1985 May;41 (5 Suppl):1132-45.

26) McDougall JA. "Vegan" "Plant-based" "Starchivore" What Do You Call Yourself? *The McDougall Newsletter*. April 2013; Vol. 12, No. 4.

27) McDougall JA. Sugar, coated with myths, we are hard wired to enjoy sugar.

The McDougall Newsletter. Sept 2006; Vol. 5, No. 9.

28) McDougall JA. The Smoke and Mirrors of Grain Brain and Wheat Belly. *The McDougall Newsletter*. Jan 2013; Vol. 13, No. 1.

29) McDougall JA. When friends ask; Where do you get your protein? *The McDougall Newsletter*. April 2007; Vol.6, No. 4.

30) Cummings J., Hill M.J., Bones E.S., Branch W.J., Jenkins D.J. The effect of meat protein and dietary fiber on colonic function and metabolism. II. Bacterial metabolites in feces and urine. *Am J Clin Nutr*. 1979;32:2094–2101.

31) Brown K, DeCoffe D, Molcan E, Gibson DL. Diet-induces

dysbiosis of the intestinal microbiota and the effects on immunity and disease. *Nutrients.* 2012 Aug; 4(8):1095-1119.

32) McDougall JA. How to help a meathead. *The McDougall Newsletter.* Nov 2003; Vol. 2, No. 11.

33) Xiao Y, Zhang Y, Wang M, Li X, Xia M, Ling W. Dietary protein and plasma total homocysteine, cysteine concentrations in coronary angiographic subjects. *Nutrition Journal.* Nov 2013;12:144 DOI:10.1186/1475-2891-12-144.

34) Campbell TC, Campbell TM. *The China Study; The most comprehensive study of nutrition ever conducted and the startling implications for diet, weight loss and long-term health.* Dallas, Texas: Benbella Books, Inc., 2006. Print.

35) Lara-Castro C, Garvey WT. Intracellular lipid accumulation in liver and muscle and the insulin resistance syndrome. *Endocrinol Metab Clin North Am.* 2008 Dec; 37(4):841-856.

36) McDougall JA. When friends ask; Where do you get your protein? *The McDougall Newsletter.* April 2007, Vol. 6, No. 4.

37) Domingo JL, Nadal M. Carcinogenicity of consumption of red meat and processed meat: A review of scientific news since the IARC decision. *Epub* 2017 Apr 24.

38) Piccoli GB, Vigoti FN, Leone F, et al. Low-protein diets in chronic kidney disease: how can we achieve them? A narrative, pragmatic review. *Clin Kidney J.* 2015;8(1): 61-70.

39) McDougall JA. When Friends Ask: Where do you get your calcium from? *The McDougall Newsletter.* Feb 2007; Vol. 6, No. 2.

40) McDougall JA. When Friends Ask: Why don't you drink milk? *The McDougall Newsletter.* March 2007; Vol. 6, No. 3.

41) Cronin J. Don't say cheese: Cheese is number one source of artery clogging fat in American diet. *Center for Science in the Public Interest.* February 2001 Article online: cspinet.org/new/cheese.html

42) McDougall JA. When Friends Ask: Why do you avoid adding vegetable oils? *The McDougall Newsletter.* Aug 2007, Vol.6, No. 8.

43) McDougall JA. Marketing milk and disease. *The McDougall Newsletter*. May 2003; Vol. 2, No. 5.

44) McDougall JA. The 2015 dietary guidelines are intended to confuse the public and press. *The McDougall Newsletter*. Feb 2015; Vol. 15, No. 2.

45) McDougall JA. Confessions of a fish killer. *The McDougall Newsletter*. June 2007; Vol. 16, No. 6.

46) Hooper L, Thompson RL, Harrison RA, Summerbell CD, Ness AR, Moore HJ, Worthington HV, Durrington PN, Higgins JP. Risks and benefits of omega 3 fats for mortality, cardiovascular disease, and cancer: systematic review. *BMJ*. 2006 Apr 1;332(7544):752-60.

47) McDougall JA. Soy-Food, Wonder drug, or poison? Calcium loss and cancer growth from protein concentrates. *The McDougall Newsletter*. April 2005; Vol. 14, No. 4.

48) Ornish D, Lin J, Chan JM, Epel E, Kemp C, et al. Effect of comprehensive lifestyle changes on telomerase activity and telomere length in men with biopsy-proven low-risk prostate cancer: 5-year follow-up of a descriptive pilot study. *The Lancet Oncology*. October 2013; Vol. 14, No. 11: p1112-1120.

49) Kapadia CR. Vitamin B_{12} in health and disease: part I – inherited disorders of function, absorption, and transport. *Gastroenterologist*. 1995 Dec; 3(4):329-44.

50) McDougall JA. Just to be on the safe side: don't take vitamins. *The McDougall Newsletter*. May 2010; Vol. 9, Issue 5.

51) McDougall JA. Plants, not pills, for vitamins and minerals. The depleted soils sales pitch. *The McDougall Newsletter*. Aug 2003; Vol. 2, No. 8.

52) McDougall JA. Adding pleasure to the satisfaction of starches: Sugar does not cause obesity or diabetes. *The McDougall Newsletter*. June 2010; Vol. 19, No. 6.

53) McDougall JA. Refined carbohydrates for food addicts: Refined sugars are empty calories and rob your body of nutrients. *The McDougall Newsletter*. Oct 2006; Vol. 5, No. 10.

54) Adams KM, Butsch WS, Kohlmeier M. The state of nutrition education at US medical schools. *Journal of Biomedical Education*. 2015, Article ID 357627, 7 pages http://dx.doi.org/1.1155/215/357627.

55) McDougall JA. SB 380 will Require Physicians to Learn about Nutrition. *The McDougall Newsletter*. Jun 2013; Vol. 12, No. 6.

56) McDougall JA. The McDougall Program under Trump's rule, Donald Trump will make a big difference but for whom? Food libel laws. *The McDougall Newsletter*. Nov 2016; Vol. 15, No. 11.

57) Heid M. Experts say lobbying skewed the U.S. dietary guidelines. *Time Health*. January 2016. Online Article: time.com/4130043/lobbying-politics-dietary-guidelines/

58) Dr McDougall's Skype Interview for the Toronto Starch Solution Meetup Group, Nov. 2016.

59) McDougall JA. Al Gore vegan diet: The power of the individual. *The McDougall Newsletter*. Nov 2013; Vol.12, No. 11.

60) HSUS Report: The welfare of animals in the meat, egg, and dairy industries. Online pdf: humanesociety.org.

61) Buff E. Can we solve world hunger and feed 9 billion people just by eating less meat? *One Green Planet*. May 2017; Online article: onegreenplanet.org/environment/world-hunger-population-growth-ditching-meat/

Chapter Four

1) White BA, Horwath CC, Conner TS. Many apples a day keep the blues away – daily experiences of negative and positive affect and food consumption in young adults. *Br J Health Psychol*. 1997;23:94-102.

2) Fraser GE. Vegetarian diets: what do we know of their effects on common chronic diseases? *Am J Clin Nutr*. May 2009; 89(5):167S-1612S.

3) Rooney C., McKinley M.C., Woodside J.V. The potential role of fruit and vegetables in aspects of psychological well-being: A review of

the literature and future directions. *Proc. Nutr. Soc.* 2013;72:420-432.

4) McDougall JA, McDougall MA. *The Starch Solution; Eat the foods you love, regain your health, and lose the weight for good!* New York, NY: Rodale, 2012. Print.

5) Sinha R, Cross AJ, Graubard BI, Leitzmann MF, Schatzkin A. Meat intake and mortality: a prospective study of over half a million people. *Arch Intern Med.* 2009 Mar 23; 169(6):562-71.

6) Subramanian S, Chait A. The effect of dietary cholesterol on macrophage accumulation in adipose tissue: implications for systemic inflammation and atherosclerosis. *Curr Opin Lipidol.* 2009 Feb;20(1):39-44.

7) Morin RJ, Hu B, Peng SK, Sevanian A. Cholesterol oxides and carcinogenesis. *J Clin Lab Anal.* 1991;5(3):219-25.

8) Frassetto L.Diet, evolution and aging--the pathophysiologic effects of the post-agricultural inversion of the potassium-to-sodium and base-to-chloride ratios in the human diet. Eur J Nutr. 2001 Oct;40(5):200-13.

9) Hooper L, Thompson RL, Harrison RA, Summerbell CD, Ness AR, Moore HJ, Worthington HV, Durrington PN, Higgins JP. Risks and benefits of omega 3 fats for mortality, cardiovascular disease, and cancer: systematic review. *BMJ.* 2006 Apr 1;332(7544):752-60.10)

10) Felton CV, Crook D, Davies MJ, Oliver MF. Dietary polyunsaturated fatty acids and composition of human aortic plaques. *Lancet.* 1994 Oct 29;344(8931):1195-6.

11) Lu M, Taylor A, Chylack LT Jr, Rogers G, Hankinson SE, Willett WC, Jacques PF. Dietary fat intake and early age-related lens opacities. *Am J Clin Nutr.* 2005 Apr;81(4):773-9.

12) Griffini P. Dietary omega-3 polyunsaturated fatty acids promote colon carcinoma metastasis in rat liver. *Cancer Res.* 1998 Aug 1;58(15):3312-9.

13) Lisle DJ, Goldhamer A. *The Pleasure Trap; Mastering the hidden force that undermines health and happiness.* Summertown, Tenessee: Healthy

Living Publications, 2003. Print.

14) Adams KM, Butsch WS, Kohlmeier M. The state of nutrition education at US medical schools. *Journal of Biomedical Education.* 2015, Article ID 357627, 7 pages http://dx.doi.org/1.1155/215/357627.

15) Kolderup A, Svihus B. Fructose metabolism and relation to atherosclerosis, type 2 diabetes, and obesity. *Journal of Nutrition and Metabolism.* Volume 2015 (2015), Article ID 823081, 12 pages. http://dx.doi.org/10.1155/2015/823081

16) Cummings J., Hill M.J., Bones E.S., Branch W.J., Jenkins D.J. The effect of meat protein and dietary fiber on colonic function and metabolism. II. Bacterial metabolites in feces and urine. *Am J Clin Nutr.* 1979;32:2094–2101.

17) Brown K, DeCoffe D, Molcan E, Gibson DL. Diet-induces dysbiosis of the intestinal microbiota and the effects on immunity and disease. *Nutrients.* 2012 Aug; 4(8):1095-1119.

18) Dewell A, Weidner G, Sumner MD, et al. Relationship of dietary protein and soy isoflavones to serum IGF-1 and IGF binding proteins in the Prostate Cancer Lifestyle Trial. *Nutr Cancer.* 2007;58:35-42.

19) Hellerstein MK, Schwarz JM, Neese RA. Regulation of hepatic de novo lipogenesis in humans. *Annu Rev Nutr.* 1996;16:523-57.

20) Northey JM, Cherbuin N, Pumpa KL, et al. Exercise interventions for cognitive function in adults older than 50: a systematic review with meta-analysis. *British Journal of Sports Medicine.* Published online April 24 2017.

21) Guure CB, Ibrahim NA, Adam MB, Said SM. Impact of physical activity on cognitive decline, dementia, and its subtypes: meta-analysis of prospective studies. *BioMed Research International.* Volume 2017 (2017), Article ID 9016924, 13 pages https://doi.org/10.1155/2017/9016924

22) Guszkowska M. Effects of exercise on anxiety, depression and mood. *Psychiatr Pol.* 2004 Jul-Aug;38(4):611-20.

23) McDougall JA, McDougall MA. *The McDougall Program for Maximum*

Weight Loss. New York, NY: Plume (Penguin Group), 1995. Print.

24) Bozian RC, Ferguson JL, Heyssel RM, Meneely GR, Darby WJ. Evidence concerning the human requirement for vitamin B_{12}. Use of the whole body counter for determination of absorption of vitamin B_{12}. *Am J Clin Nutr.* 1963;12:117–129.

25) Kon S. XXXV. The value of whole potato in human nutrition. *Biochemical J.* 1928; 2:258-260.

Resources

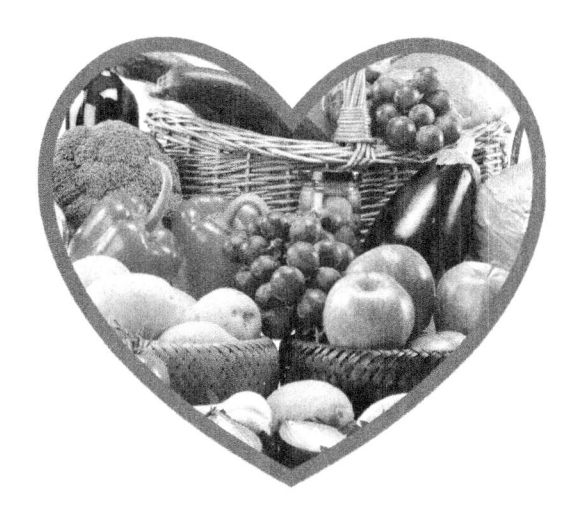

Experts, Doctors, Dietitians, Books, Articles, Youtube Channels, Websites, Movies, Products and Services

Toronto Starch Solution Meetup Group
Group Toronto Starch Solution Meetup

Resources

Additional help to get you started and keep you going.

Online Resources

Dr. John McDougall's website: https://www.drmcdougall.com/

Mary McDougall's recipes: https://www.drmcdougall.com/health/education/recipes/

The Toronto Starch Solution Meetup Group: https://www.meetup.com/Toronto-Starch-Solution-Meetup/

Susan Voisin's Fat Free Kitchen: http://blog.fatfreevegan.comu

Dana's Minimalist Baker: http://blog.fatfreevegan.com

Chuck Underwood's Brand New Vegan: http://www.brandnewvegan.com

Cathy Fisher's Straight Up Food: http://www.straightupfood.com/blog/

Katie Mae's Plantz Street: https://plantzst.com

Dreena Burton's Plant Powered Kitchen: http://plantpoweredkitchen.com

Lindsay Nixon's Happy Herbivore: https://happyherbivore.com

Chef Del Sroufe: http://chefdelsroufe.com/recipes/

Jeff Novick, RD: http://www.jeffnovick.com/RD/Home.html

Dr. Michael Greger's Nutrition Facts website: https://nutritionfacts.org/

Dr. Caldwell Esselstyn's website: http://www.dresselstyn.com/site/

Dr. T. Colin Campbell's website: http://nutritionstudies.org/

Dr. Neal Barnard, Physician's Committee for Responsible Medicine: http://www.pcrm.org/media/experts/neal-barnard

Dr. Michael Klaper's website: http://doctorklaper.com/

Brenda Davis, RD: http://www.brendadavisrd.com/

Dr. Pamela Popper's website: http://drpampopper.com/

Chef AJ's website: http://chefajwebsite.com/index.html

TrueNorth Health Center: http://www.healthpromoting.com/

John Pierre: http://www.johnpierre.com/

Dr. Richard Oppenlander's website: http://comfortablyunaware.com/

Dr. Doug Lisle - Esteem Dynamics: http://esteemdynamics.org/

Julianna Hever, RD: http://plantbaseddietitian.com/about/

Lindsay Nixon : http://happyherbivore.com

Books

The Starch Solution by John A. McDougall, MD and Mary McDougall

The McDougall Program for Maximum Weight Loss by John A. McDougall, MD and Mary McDougall

The Healthiest Diet on the Planet by John A. McDougall, MD and Mary

McDougall

The China Study by T. Colin Campbell, PhD, and Thomas M. Campbell II, MD

Whole by T. Colin Campbell, PhD, and with Howard Jacobson, PhD

How Not to Die by Michael Greger, MD

Prevent and Reverse Heart Disease by Caldwell Esselstyn, Jr., MD

The Pleasure Trap by Douglas J. Lisle, PhD and Alan Goldhamer, DC

Comfortably Unaware by Richard Oppenlander, DDS

Films

Forks over Knives

Cowspiracy: The Sustainability Secret

What The Health

Plant Pure Nation

Eating You Alive

Food Inc.

Earthlings

Vegucated

Live and Let Live

Okja

We want to hear from you!

If you have found success with this way of eating and living, please tell us your stories! We'd love to hear from you. Just email us at the address below.

Contact the Authors

If you or your organization are interested in hiring the authors for speaking engagements or workshops, please contact us at:

fedupwithbeingfatandsick @ gmail dot **com**

Need some help?

Hi, I'm Judith Fiore. I'm a licensed naturopathic doctor and I'm available for consultation if you need extra help getting started on the nutritional plan that you've read about in this book.

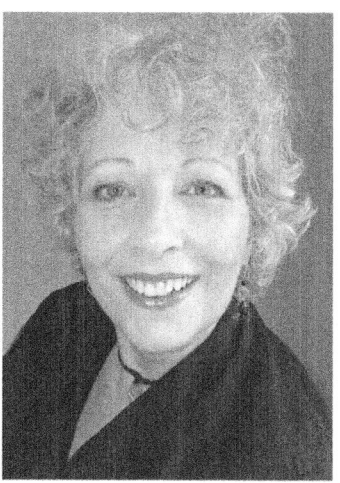

**Judith Fiore, B.A. (Psychology)
N.D. (Doctor of Naturopathic Medicine)**

I can help you with planning your meals, shopping, trips to restaurants, social events, dealing with loved ones who may be sabotaging your efforts, and anything else that is a challenge for you.

For those of you who are living with issues that aren't completely addressed by folowing The Starch Solution plan, a naturopathic consultation will help you to make additional changes to improve your health and well-being.

You can reach me through my website:
www.drjudithfiore.com

Jump for Joy
VEGAN GIFTS

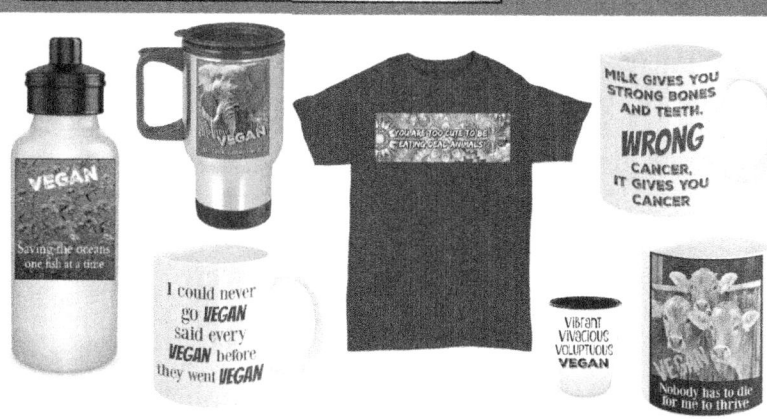

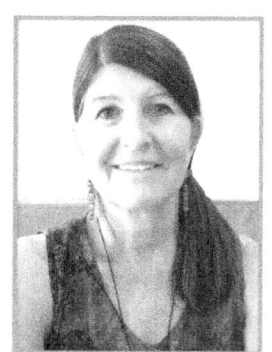

Hi, this is Diane McConnell. As you travel further down the path to better health with this nutritional lifestyle, consider these products for your own enjoyment or to share with family and friends. Tell the world what you have done to change your life for the better. Celebrate your success!

I have created these products: t-shirts, reusable water bottles, coffee cups, and travel mugs with vegan messages. These are conversation starters. They also show you care about something important. The more people see these messages, the more main stream they become. Together we spreading the word about the power of a whole food plant-based diet, not only to regain optimal health, but to help the animals and heal the Earth. My designs are available on both Amazon and Etsy.

Place your order now!

Amazon	Etsy
http://bit.ly/mugsbyrodm	http://bit.ly/veganjoygifts

Help spread the word!

Write us a review!

If you have been inspired by the stories in this book, we invite you to share your experience with others. The more people who write a review, the more likely this valuable information will be able to get out and help improve lives.

Printed in Great Britain
by Amazon